THE **PALEO** DIET SOLUTION

JOHN CHATHAM

D1716585

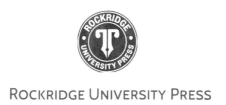

ROCKRIDGE UNIVERSITY PRESS

THE PALEO DIET SOLUTION

THE **PALEO** DIET SOLUTION

SECTION ONE

An Introduction to the Paleo Diet

CHAPTER 1

What is the Paleo Diet?

The Paleo or Paleolithic Diet goes by several names. It's also commonly called the Stone Age Diet, the Caveman Diet or the Hunter-Gatherer Diet. Regardless of the name used, it is a diet based on what is known and what is assumed about the daily diet of man prior to the age of agriculture. The diet gets its most common title from the age known as the Paleolithic Era, a time that spanned from about 2.5 million years ago to about 10,000 years ago, when man started to grow crops as a source of food.

The Paleo Diet guidelines are based on a pattern of eating that attempts to replicate, as closely as is possible in modern times, a diet based on foods that could have been hunted, fished or foraged in the wild during this pre-agricultural age. These foods include wild game, meats, fish and shellfish, eggs, fruits and vegetables, mushrooms, tree nuts, seeds, herbs and honey.

There are several variations of the Paleo Diet, which differ in how strictly they adhere to the most stringent guidelines. The original Paleo Diet excludes all grains, dairy, legumes (beans) and sugar. Some more flexible versions allow for a very limited amount of grains, legumes or dairy, but most versions either exclude them completely or only allow them in the very smallest quantities.

All variations of the Paleo Diet forbid any processed foods, alcohol or sugar.

The premise behind the Paleo Diet is the theory that we are not genetically wired to process foods such as legumes, grains and dairy and that many of the health issues we face today are a result of eating foods to which our bodies are not truly adapted. These health issues, such as obesity, diabetes and heart disease, are often referred to as "diseases of affluence." This is because they are most common, and even considered epidemic, in the wealthier nations, where people eat rich diets far removed from the land.

The creators of the various versions of the Paleo Diet claim that many of these nutrition-related diseases can be avoided or aided by following this pattern of eating. A good deal of research supports this claim. As a side benefit, the Paleo Diet can also help followers to lose weight, although its main purpose is good health; primarily good cardiovascular health and a stronger immune system.

The Paleo Diet does require commitment and creativity, as it means giving up many of the foods and ingredients that most Americans are used to eating on a daily basis. Adjusting to this pattern of eating and finding suitable substitutes for off-limit foods can take some time and a good deal of trial and error. However, the benefits to your health, weight and feeling of wellbeing make that time and effort well worthwhile.

CHAPTER 2

How the Paleo Diet Came About

The Paleo Diet has become enormously popular in the last few years and has garnered quite a bit of media attention. However, the Paleo Diet is far from a newcomer to the nutrition/diet arena. In fact, it's more than thirty years old.

The Beginning of a New Way to Eat

In 1975, gastroenterologist Walter L. Voegtlin published his book, The Stone Age Diet, in which he presented a convincing case for returning to a diet more like that followed by peoples of the Paleolithic Era. In the book, Dr. Voegtlin presented several examples of his treatment of digestive ailments such as colitis, irritable bowel syndrome and Crohn's disease with a diet that relied primarily on animal fats and proteins and a very low intake of carbohydrates.

In the 70's, it was almost universally believed that the only healthy diet was one that was low in fat and calories, so the Stone Age Diet didn't make much of an impact on mainstream thought.

The Caveman Goes Mainstream

In 1985, however, Boyd Eaton and Melvin Konner, of Emory University, published an article in The New England Journal of Medicine that did gain a great deal of attention in both the media and the public. Their paper was a study of Paleolithic nutrition that led to the 1988 release of their book, The Paleolithic Prescription: A Program of Diet & Exercise and a Design for Living. This book became the foundation for today's many variations of the Paleo Diet.

The Paleo Diet Solution

In the book, the authors explained the components and benefits of the Paleolithic Era diet, although their recommendation was to reproduce the pattern and macronutrient content of the diet using modern foods, rather than excluding any foods that would not have been available to people of the Stone Age. This book was quickly followed by their second book, The Stone Age Health Programme, which presented more research about the health benefits of eating the way our ancestors ate.

CHAPTER 3

What the Paleo Diet Can Do for Your Health

Many people choose to follow the Paleo Diet because they want a safe, effective and pleasant way to lose weight. However, the Paleo Diet is much more than a weight loss diet; it's a new approach to nutrition and eating that can provide enormous benefits to your health.

The Paleo Diet and Heart Health

The Paleo Diet's impact on heart or cardiovascular health is responsible for much of the attention that's been focused on the diet. It's easy to understand the confusion that some people have over claims that a diet high in animal protein can actually make your heart healthier. We've been conditioned to think that animal protein equals fat and fat equals bad for your heart.

The truth is that we now know that the animal protein eaten by our Paleolithic ancestors was much, much lower in saturated fat than the animal protein we consume today. It was also much higher in heart-healthy Omega 3 fatty acids, which we know are incredibly beneficial not only to our hearts, but also our brain function and immune systems. A diet high in these healthy fats will also aid considerably in weight loss, particularly abdominal fat loss. Abdomen fat and a thick waistline are known to be markers of future heart disease.

The Paleo Diet is based on animal proteins that are low in saturated fats yet high in Omega 3 fatty acids – these are grass fed livestock animals, free-range or wild poultry and pork, wild game animals and birds and fish, shellfish and mollusks.

This menu of animal proteins is much lower in saturated fats and much higher in healthy fats, which reduces abdominal fat, can prevent, reduce or reverse arterial disease, and lowers unhealthy LDL cholesterol while raising healthier HDL cholesterol.

The Paleo Diet and Diabetes, Pre-Diabetes and Metabolic Syndrome

Type 2 diabetes has reached epidemic proportions in the US and other Western cultures. The predominance of processed foods, white flour and sugar in our daily diets is being blamed for much of the type 2 diabetes we're suffering in this country, as well as for the millions of people who are diagnosed with metabolic syndrome (the predecessor of diabetes).

> *Did you know? Sweden's Lund University recently conducted a landmark study comparing the effects of a healthy Western diet versus the Paleo Diet. In the study, 19 men with diabetes or pre-diabetes followed each diet for three months. The results showed that the men on the Paleo Diet improved their glucose tolerance by 26%, versus a 7% improvement on the Western diet.*

The Paleo Diet is a high-protein/low carbohydrate diet that focuses on low-glycemic carbs and is completely free of processed foods, wheat flours and sugar. Because of this, people with diabetes, pre-diabetes or metabolic syndrome are able to reduce blood sugar levels, maintain healthy levels and increase insulin sensitivity. Additionally, the Paleo Diet aids in reducing abdominal fat, which is one of the top priorities for anyone with diabetes or metabolic syndrome.

The Paleo Diet and Digestive Issues

One of the most important premises of the Paleo Diet is that for 99.6% of our history of 2.5 million years, we consumed no grains or legumes. As a result, the last

10,000 years has not been enough time for our genetics to adapt to the consumption of these foods. Researchers believe that it is this lack of adaptation that has created so many digestive disorders in Westerners, including colitis, irritable bowel syndrome and many others. Many scientists and nutritionists also believe that abstaining from grains and legumes and eating plenty of plant fiber can guard colon health and may even prevent many cases of colon cancer. Many followers report fewer incidences of less severe digestive issues, such as constipation, heartburn, acid reflux and excess gas.

The Paleo Diet and Your Immune System

Following the Paleo Diet can have just as great an effect on your immune system and any auto-immune disorders as it does on digestive and heart disorders. Many researchers and medical experts blame the consumption of foods such as grains, legumes and dairy, which our bodies have not adapted to, for creating overactive immune systems in many westerners.

Because we are not adapted to eating these foods, our immune systems see them as allergens or outsiders, whether we experience any "allergic reactions" or not. A high intake of these foods causes our immune system to become overactive, which increases inflammation in many different cells in tissues.

In 2011, French doctor Jean Seignalet conducted a study involving hundreds of patients with such immune disorders as Lupus, rheumatoid arthritis, fibromyalgia and multiple sclerosis, among others. The patients involved followed a raw/lightly cooked Paleo Diet with incredible results. Dr. Seignalet's yardstick was a 50% reduction in symptoms and severity. At the end of the study, the number of patients who reached this goal were:

Rheumatoid Arthritis...................80%
Lupus..100%
Fibromyalgia.............................97%
Multiple Sclerosis.....................97%

Dr. Seignalet's study supports the theory behind the Paleo Diet: that eliminating foods we are not genetically adapted to eating will greatly reduce many diseases, disorders and health issues.

With so many of our systems and so many huge health problems showing dramatic improvement on the Paleo Diet, it's easy to see why so many in the scientific and medical communities are excited about adopting this healthier, more natural way of eating.

CHAPTER 4

The Paleo Diet and Allergies

One of the most exciting things about the Paleo Diet is that it's a wonderful way of cutting out common allergens in our foods. As we've said, many respected researchers and scientists feel that dairy, grains and legumes are not foods that we are genetically adapted to; therefore, they create or contribute to many common and serious health problems. The Paleo Diet is also a great diet for those who have known allergies to dairy and grains, because these foods are eliminated from the diet altogether.

The Paleo Diet and Celiac Disease

Because grains and legumes are eliminated from the diet, the Paleo Diet is a great diet for those with Celiac disease or sensitivity to gluten.

Celiac disease is being diagnosed in increasingly higher numbers today. The American diet is filled with wheat products such as breads, pastries, pancakes, muffins, cookies and even gravies, sauces, and crackers. Those with Celiac disease or sensitivity to gluten or wheat have a very tough time trying to find foods they can eat safely.

The Paleo Diet is a naturally gluten-free diet, yet provides plenty of fiber and carbohydrates through plant foods. Many followers of the diet are even able to enjoy some of their favorite foods, substituting various nut flours and other ingredients for the wheat flour they traditionally include.

The Paleo Diet and Lactose Intolerance

More and more Americans are discovering that their various digestive issues are a result of an intolerance of or sensitivity to cow's milk and sometimes even goat's milk. Problems such as bloating, cramping, excess gas, nausea and diarrhea are a result of their body's inability to digest these dairy products.

Because the Paleo Diet excludes all dairy products, it's an easy one to adopt for those on a dairy-free diet or who are thinking about removing dairy from their lives.

While many people with lactose intolerance switch to drinking lactose-free alternatives such as soy milk, the Paleo Diet doesn't allow soy, as soybeans are a legume. This is why many people with lactose issues may still experience digestive and other symptoms, even when drinking soy milk and eating other soy products.

Followers of the Paleo Diet often substitute healthier nut milks such as coconut or almond milk, which can be used both for drinking and for cooking and baking.

The Paleo Diet and Other Allergy Issues

In addition to these two prevalent allergy issues, much of the discomfort or illness we experience may come from the additives in our foods, including antibiotics, hormones and preservatives.

By eliminating processed foods and choosing organic, grass fed and free-range plant and animal foods, you can avoid virtually all of these harmful and often hidden ingredients.

Many people who are unaware of any particular food allergies report that after a few months on the Paleo Diet, they notice much less inflammation, fewer headaches and much less stomach upset. This unexpected result supports the idea that we are all allergic to these foods because our genetics have not adapted us to eating them.

Did you know? As you follow the Paleo Diet for the first several weeks, keep a small notebook handy to track any improvement in conditions such as heartburn, acid reflux, constipation, diarrhea, frequent headaches, nausea and any other ongoing health problems. Schedule an appointment with your doctor to discuss these changes; you may be able to reduce or eliminate costly and possibly harmful medications.

CHAPTER 5

The Paleo Diet and Weight Loss

Although the health benefits of following the Paleo Diet are clear and important, many people are primarily interested in using the Paleo Diet to help them lose weight. The good news is that you can lose weight quite easily on the Paleo Diet and reap the health benefits while you're at it.

At first glance, many people may think that the Paleo Diet doesn't seem like a way to lose weight. We're so conditioned to think that cutting back on meats and taking in more high-fiber grains and cereals are two key ways to lose weight. However, the Paleo Diet will help you to lose weight effectively, healthfully and without the hunger pangs we've come to expect from dieting.

There are several reasons why the Paleo Diet works so well to help you lose weight:

- High quality proteins help to build muscle and ward off hunger.

- Omega 3 fatty acids help to reduce body fat.

- High content of Vitamin C helps to metabolize fat.

- High fiber from plant sources keeps digestion efficient.

- Low-sugar diet aids in increasing insulin resistance.

- Low-glycemic carbs from plant foods keeps energy high and hunger at bay.

Let's take a look at each of these components of the Paleo Diet and how they help you to lose weight.

High Quality Animal and Seafood Proteins

Many experts recommend that approximately 60%-70% of your daily diet comes from high-quality lean meats and seafood.

Protein is essential for muscle growth and function as well as cell-building and brain function. Protein also helps you to lose weight by satisfying your hunger longer than any other macronutrient. Protein is metabolized much more slowly than carbs, so it remains in your stomach longer, providing a feeling of satisfaction or satiety. The fats in meats also help to keep you feeling fuller longer.

Protein is also essential for helping you to build lean muscle. When you accompany the diet with a moderate amount of resistance training, you'll see rapid changes in the shape of your body. In just a few weeks, you'll begin to see longer, leaner muscles, flatter abdominals and a smaller waistline.

Omega 3 Fatty Acids

Omega 3 fatty acids are the superheroes of the micronutrients. They increase heart health, improve memory, reduce depression and even help you to lose stubborn fat deposits, particularly around the abdomen.

Omega 3 fatty acids are called essential fatty acids because we don't naturally produce them in our bodies; we must get them from our diet. Among the many ways our body uses Omega 3 fatty acids is in the production of eicosanoids-hormones that regulate insulin production, digestion and the storage of fat.

Getting plenty of Omega 3 fatty acids in your diet ensures that your body produces enough eicosanoids for all of your body's needs.

Insulin production will increase, helping your body to metabolize glucose into glycogen so that it can be used for energy instead of stored as fat.

Did you know? A recent study placed half of its subjects on a diet supplemented with fish oil supplements rich in Omega 3 fatty acids. The other half of the research group was placed on the same diet without the Omega 3 supplementation. At the end of the study, the group taking Omega 3 supplements had 50% lower blood insulin levels and lost 26% more body fat than the people who did not take the supplements.

Vitamin C

In the 1985 New England Journal of Medicine article, Eaton & Konner reported their somewhat surprising finding that Paleolithic man's diet was enormously richer in Vitamin C than the average diet today. This is mainly because they ate a great deal of plant foods and ate them at the peak of freshness, as soon as they were picked or very shortly thereafter.

Even those of us who eat a great deal of produce often eat many fruits and vegetables out of season, after they've been shipped thousands of miles. They've already lost a great deal of the vitamin content before they've reached us, particularly their Vitamin C.

Vitamin C is enormously valuable in the area of weight loss. Its two most important contributions are the production of L-carnitine and the reduction in the amount of cortisol released into our bloodstreams.

L-Carnitine is a compound created by the body from certain amino acids. During the breakdown of fats, L-Carnitine's role is to transport fatty acids to the mitochondria so that they can be used (or burned) as energy.

Research shows that Vitamin C is essential for the production of L-Carnitine and that without sufficient L-Carnitine, the body's ability to burn stored fat as energy will be dramatically slowed.

The Paleo Diet helps you to burn not only the fats that you eat, but the fat that you already have stored on your body!

Vitamin C and Cortisol

Cortisol has gotten plenty of attention in the media today, particularly in health magazines and diet and weight loss books. If you missed the news or need a refresher course, cortisol is one of the body's stress hormones. The stress hormones have several jobs, but cortisol's job is to direct the storage or disposal of fat around the abdomen. When the body's perceives a time of stress, more cortisol is released to the bloodstream and that cortisol signals the need to store fat on the abdomen in case of famine in the near future. This age-old reaction was created because the fight or flight system in our bodies was meant to not only help us hurry to safety, but to survive a food shortage until we got there.

This is a great system, but it usually works against us today, when stress rarely signals a food shortage or a need to be on the run without time to hunt or gather. Most of us live stress-filled lives as a rule and even everyday stress such as that caused by tight schedules, family issues or a job change can bring about a surge in the amount of cortisol running through our bodies.

> *Did you know?* A recent research study found that even the stress of counting calories while on a diet will cause more cortisol to be released into the bloodstream. In the study, subjects were put on the same 1600 calorie diet, but half of the subjects had their food chosen for them while the other half had to divvy up their 1600 calories each day. At the end of the study, the subjects who had no need to count calories had lost more body fat! The good part of this? On the Paleo Diet, calorie counting is strongly discouraged!!

So where does Vitamin C come in to the cortisol effect? Vitamin C reduces the effects of stress on the body. Vitamin C is a soluble vitamin – we're not able to store much of it at once. Stress depletes the body's stores at a rapid rate, and that drop in Vitamin C, which is needed by every cell in our bodies, is one of the warning signals the body uses to detect stress.

By eating a diet very high in Vitamin C, like the Paleo Diet, you can slow the production and release of cortisol and up your production of L-Carnitine. In short, you'll store less new body fat and burn more of the fat you already have stored up. That is a dieter's win-win situation.

High Fiber

There are two types of dietary fiber: soluble and insoluble. Both are essential to good health and each is equally important to those trying to lose weight. Fortunately, even though grains are excluded from the Paleo Diet, the diet is rich in the best source of these two types of fiber-plant foods.

Soluble fiber dissolves in water during digestion. When it does, it becomes a gel-like substance that gives us a feeling of fullness and also slows the absorption of sugar into the blood. Insoluble fiber is completely indigestible – it passes through the digestive system in almost the same state it was in when you ate it. The importance of insoluble fiber is that it speeds waste through the digestive tract and cleans the colon as it does so. An efficient digestive system helps you to rid your body of built-up toxins, fats and other unwelcome hangers-on.

The best source of these two fibers is plant foods. While higher concentrations are found in the bran covering of whole grains, the fiber content of plants comes with more vitamins, minerals and other essential micronutrients.

Your fiber-rich Paleo Diet helps you to lose weight more quickly and healthfully by improving and speeding up digestion, slowing the absorption of fat and carbs and helping you to feel satisfied longer.

No Sugar/Low Glycemic Diet

The Paleo Diet excludes all refined sugars and syrups and all grains, so it is naturally sugar free and contains a very low glycemic load. Unless you're a diabetic, you won't need to limit yourself to fruits and veggies with a low-glycemic index, as the overall glycemic load of your meals and snacks will be very low.

The importance of this is two-fold: The lack of sugar in your diet will soon "reset" your body's insulin resistance, making your system much more sensitive to insulin and lowering your blood glucose levels. The low glycemic load will prevent blood sugar spikes and drops, keeping cravings and hunger at bay while providing you with a steady source of energy.

Another related benefit is that by removing sugar and a great deal of the simple carbs (flours and refined foods) from your diet, you will help your body to start using the protein in your diet as energy. Contrary to what some diet books will tell you, the body can use any type of food for energy; however, it uses the easiest sources first. Sugar and other carbohydrates convert to glucose more easily, so the body will use them first. Once those stores are depleted, it will begin to convert proteins and then fats.

One of the reasons that cavemen remained lean and were also able to run ten miles while hunting food, without carbing up first, is that their bodies were efficient at converting protein and fat to energy. Once you've been on the Paleo Diet for a few weeks, your body will start doing this, too.

As you can see, there are plenty of reasons to be excited about following the Paleo Diet in order to lose weight. You'll be eating foods that speed weight loss, you won't have to count calories and you'll be eating a daily diet that helps you to feel full, not hungry and deprived.

Did you know? Most people will lose weight on the first few weeks of the Paleo Diet simply because of the foods they won't be eating. If you still have weight to lose after the first month or so, cut back on portions, but keep your protein intake at the recommended percentages, getting most of it from lower-calorie seafood and eggs. Once you've reached your desired weight, add more animal proteins and up your portion sizes to maintain your weight.

CHAPTER 6

The Paleo Diet for Athletes

M any athletes involved in strength-training and muscle building sports were quick to jump on board with the Paleo Diet, as most of them were already following a high-protein, low-carb eating plan. However, endurance athletes, such as long distance runners, cyclists and swimmers were a little dubious at first. Endurance athletes have been conditioned for decades to eat a high-carb diet filled with pastas, breads and cereals and to "carb-up" or really pack on the carbs in the hours before an athletic event, such as a marathon. The Paleo Diet seemed to fly in the face of that thinking.

A New Way of Eating for Athletes

Endurance athletes got a new view of the Paleo Diet with the release of The Paleo Diet for Athletes: A Nutritional Formula for Peak Athletic Performance, written by exercise physiologist Loren Cordain, PhD. (His co-author, Joe Friel, is a triathlete and coach.) Dr. Cordain is a former marathoner and is still a fitness runner. He was intrigued by Eaton and Konner's paper in The New England Journal of Medicine and started doing his own research to learn how people (both Paleolithic man and several tribes today that follow the same basic diet) on such a low-carb diet could engage in distance running on a regular basis.

Cordain was fascinated by the rather remarkable fact that Paleolithic man got 55% of his daily calories from meat and yet had no trouble running as many as ten miles to catch his dinner. This fact led to a great deal of research into how and why the body uses protein for energy and how the Paleo Diet can help our modern bodies do the same thing.

Like Drs. Eaton and Konner, Cordain concluded that the grains most endurance athletes depend on were "man's original fast food – cheap, easy to obtain, overly processed and actually not that good for you."

In his book, Cordain answers the concerns raised by many that a diet without grains would be deficient in many nutrients. His reply: "Grains can't hold a micronutrient candle to fruits and vegetables."

Dr. Cordain's co-author, Joe Friel, was extremely skeptical about the Paleo Diet when they first started discussing it in the 1990s. He was convinced that the traditional pasta and cereal diet of endurance athletes was the only way to go. In fact, he went on the Paleo Diet just to prove a point to Cordain.

As he explains it, he felt lousy for the first two weeks, but in the third week he started feeling better and was able to increase his training by 50%. In the fourth week, he increased it by 50% again and has been following the Paleo Diet since then, as well as recommending it to the endurance athletes he coaches.

Naturally, the high-protein/low carb aspect of the Paleo Diet makes it an easy choice for strength-related athletes, but now endurance athletes can understand how to make the Paleo Diet work towards cardio-endurance as much as it does toward a healthy body.

Suggested Guidelines for Paleo Athletes

Dr. Cordain and others have several suggestions for maximizing performance on the Paleo Diet.

For strength-related athletes, it's recommended that athletes have a high-protein meal with a limited amount of fruits and veggies about an hour before working out, followed by a fruit snack about fifteen to thirty minutes prior to exercising. This should be followed by another high-protein meal no more than thirty minutes after working out.

For endurance athletes, such as marathoners, triathletes and long-distance cyclists, Dr. Cordain suggests a different approach; one that temporarily deviates from the normal Paleo Diet. As he says in his book,

"Training for endurance sports such as running, cycling, triathlon, rowing, swimming, and cross-country skiing places great demands on the body, and the athlete is in some stage of recovery almost continuously during periods of heavy training. The keys to optimum recovery are sleep and diet.

"Even though we recommend that everyone eat a diet similar to what our Stone Age ancestors ate, we realize that nutritional concessions must be made for the athlete who is training at a high volume (in the range of 10 to 35 or more hours per week of rigorous exercise).

Rapid recovery is the biggest issue facing such an athlete. While it's not impossible to recover from such training loads on a strict Paleo Diet, it is somewhat more difficult to recover quickly. By modifying the diet before, during, and immediately following challenging workouts, the Paleo Diet provides two benefits sought by all athletes: quick recovery for the next workout, and superior health for the rest of your life."

His recommendation follows a five-stage eating plan for endurance athletes, which we'll summarize here:

Stage One: A meal of low-glycemic carbs two hours prior to a workout or event.

Stage Two: During workouts lasting more than one hour, take 200-400 calories per hour from sports drinks.

Stage Three: In the first 30 minutes after working out intensely, drink a commercial or homemade high-carb recovery drink.

Stage Four: For the next few hours, continue to focus on high-glycemic carbs, such as sweet potatoes, yams, raisins, etc.

Stage Five: Return to the Paleo Diet until the next intense workout or endurance event.

If you're a strength-trainer, you'll probably have little trouble adapting to the Paleo Diet, as you're likely already used to a high-protein/low-carb eating plan. If you're an endurance athlete, give your body a couple of weeks to adjust, during which time you may have to cut back on training or transition more slowly to the Paleo lifestyle.

CHAPTER 7

What About All That Fat?

Many people who don't know much about the Paleo Diet or why it works are concerned with the amount of animal protein on the diet. We've been told for years that meats contain far too much saturated fat for healthy hearts and healthy waistlines. This is a valid concern and one we'll address here in simple terms that don't require degrees in chemical biology.

Why Cavemen Didn't Get Fat from All Those Steaks

Paleolithic man did indeed eat a lot of meat. It's estimated that as much as 55% of his daily caloric intake was from animal protein. However, we now know that the meat the Paleo men and women ate was free-range, grass fed and much lower in saturated fats than the meats we commonly eat today.

To replicate the quality of the animal protein in the Paleolithic diet, it's important to understand the difference between the meats we most commonly eat today and the meats we should be eating.

Most commercially available meats available at your supermarket are grain-fed, greatly increasing the amount of saturated fats in the cuts of meat you purchase. They are also filled with hormones, antibiotics and even the pesticides used on the grain that cow or pig has been fed.

The Paleo Diet stresses the importance of choosin fed, organic and free-range beef, pork and poultry, as well as wild game. These meats will not only be free of harmful chemicals but also much lower in unhealthy fats and much higher in Omega 3 fats.

Not Your Typical High-Protein Diet

Some people confuse the Paleo Diet with other popular high-protein diets, such as the original Atkins Diet. However, these diets encouraged the consumption of fatty, commercial meat products such as bacon, sausage, lunch meats and fatty cuts of beef, pork and lamb.

While some versions of the Paleo Diet make no distinction between the cuts of meat allowed, the more widely accepted guidelines (and the ones we'll use) call for leaner cuts of meat and ,again, grass fed, organic, free-range meats and wild game.

Your overall fat intake on the Paleo Diet may increase, but it will be an increase in healthy fats and a decrease in unhealthy fats. This makes all the difference in the world. *It's important to focus on the types of fat you're eating, not the number of fat grams.*

Getting Started on the Paleo Diet

CHAPTER 8

Everything You Need to Successfully Follow the Paleo Diet

Now that you have some understanding of the background, science and benefits of the Paleo Diet, it's time to get into some practical information and get you started on the way to a healthier lifestyle and a new way of eating.

There are several variations of the Paleo Diet and, in this section, we'll discuss the differences between them and why we've chosen to recommend a version that we think is more feasible and more healthful than other diets that are either quite extreme or not extreme enough.

We'll get into the guidelines of this version of the Paleo Diet and tell you all about what you'll be eating and how your daily diet will look. When you're done with this section, you'll understand what your meals will look like, how to make substitutions for grains and sugar, where to get your food and what foods you're allowed to eat. (We discuss the food guidelines here, but in the included Paleo Diet Solution Shopping Guide, you'll find a handy shopping list and supermarket guide that you can copy and take with you as you do your grocery shopping.)

We'll also give you some tips and guidelines for transitioning from a western diet to a Paleo way of eating. Use them – they'll make the first few weeks much easier and greatly increase your chances of successfully following the diet.

Paleolithic men and women were not sedentary people; they hunted, they fished, they trapped and they ran from enemies and predators. In this section, we'll discuss exercise and physical activity on the Paleo Diet and how you can use the diet to supplement your current workouts or incorporate working out into your new lifestyle.

You can find many books and guides to the Paleo Diet, but we've condensed the information down to what you really need to know to get started on and succeed with the Paleo Diet.

CHAPTER 9

The Many Variations of the Paleo Diet

Since the 1970s, many different versions and variations of the Paleo Diet have been presented to the public. It can be confusing for the beginner to figure out what is absolutely necessary and what isn't. Many people wonder, "Which is the real Paleo Diet?" The answer is, they're all real, but not every version is right for everyone. The different versions of the Paleo Diet range from what we'll call "extreme" versions to what are basically just balanced diets that call themselves Paleo Diets but miss many of the important factors that make the Paleo Diet so good for you.

Extreme Makeover: Caveman Edition

There are a few versions that will have you believe you need to actually be a hunter-gatherer, not just replicate the Paleo pattern of eating. These versions will have you feeling guilty if your meat comes wrapped in plastic or your veggies don't have dirt on them. These most extreme versions of the Paleo Diet allow for only fruits and veggies commonly found growing wild, such as watercress, asparagus, herbs, mushrooms and wild onions. While there's certainly nothing wrong with hunting wild game or scouring the forests for wild greens, this simply isn't an option for most people. If you can do some of these things and include some of these foods (and you want to), by all means do, but it certainly isn't essential to the Paleo Diet.

Call It Paleo and Sell It

At the other end of the spectrum are diets with various names that include references to Paleo, the Stone-Age or cavemen, but they're nothing more than your average balanced diet with possibly a higher protein intake than most. While they aren't unhealthy, they aren't a Paleo Diet, either. These diets don't take into consideration the proper ratio of protein to carbs, the quality of animal protein, the types of fats that should be eaten or anything else integral to the health benefits of a Paleo way of eating.

The Middle Ground

And then you have a more moderate, feasible approach that utilizes all that is healthy about the Paleo Diet while making it accessible to the modern, usually urban or suburban man and woman. This approach replicates the eating pattern and nutrient intake of Paleo peoples using foods that are commonly available to the woman with three kids and a fulltime job or the man with a demanding career and an apartment in the city. No club necessary.

This is our approach to the Paleo Diet and we feel it is the best choice for most people. No matter how healthy it is, no diet will work if you can't follow it.

CHAPTER 10

YOUR Paleo Diet: The Paleo Diet for Real People

Now that you're ready to begin the Paleo Diet, we'll get into the nuts and bolts of eating like your ancestors in a modern world. While the diet may seem somewhat restrictive in some ways because of the whole food groups that are off-limits, there are also some freedoms with the Paleo Diet.

Just Stop It!

First of all, there is no calorie counting or portioning. We really recommend that you skip all the weighing, counting and note-taking of every morsel that goes into your mouth. The Paleo Diet is a natural way of eating that your body was genetically designed to follow. The truth is, Paleo man took in a higher number of calories (and fat grams) than most diets allow. It may take some time for you to adjust your thinking about calories, but change your actions in the meantime. Once you see the results, calorie counting will no longer be a part of your mindset.

On the Paleo Diet, you'll feel more satisfied due to the increase in healthy fats, lean protein and fiber. If you follow your body's signals, you'll eat what you need rather than eating mindlessly or overeating.

The Proper Ratio of Protein to Carbs

You may think it's contradictory to tell you to take in the proper ratio of protein and carbs if you're not counting calories or grams, but the way to do it is by looking at your daily diet, your menu and your plate. If you really have a hard time gauging the ratio of protein to carbs, then go ahead and keep track of the grams you're eating for a week or so, and then you should be able to estimate the ratios without counting.

The best way to divide up your daily intake is to base each snack on a bit of protein plus a carb such as a piece of fruit. For your main meals, at least half your plate should be protein and half or less should be fruits, veggies, nuts and seeds.

Recommendations vary between different versions of the Paleo Diet, but in general your daily diet should be between 55%-65% protein, 40-30% carbs and 5% non-animal fats such as those in nuts, seeds, avocadoes and olive oil. How your diet ends up being divided is individual to your needs. Start with 55% protein and 40% carbs and if you still feel your energy level is too low after a few weeks, increase the carbs. If you find yourself grazing all day and still hungry, increase the protein.

Did you know? It will take a few weeks for your body to adjust the way it converts your food into energy. For a while, your metabolism will be waiting for that donut, whole wheat toast or bowl of granola. It's normal and expected that your energy level may be lower for the first couple of weeks, but it should increase dramatically after that, as your body starts utilizing protein for energy more efficiently.

Planning Your Daily Diet

Some versions of the Paleo Diet encourage intermittent fasting. This is based largely on findings of modern researchers, who studied several modern tribes that still eat a hunter-gatherer or Paleo-type diet. In this research, it was found that many of these tribes will often go on morning hunts that involve miles of running, without benefit of eating a morning meal.

Because of this finding, some Paleo experts recommend going long periods (ranging from several hours to a day or two) without eating. However, we think it's important to note that these tribespeople have been eating a Paleo Diet all of their lives, as did their parents, grandparents, et cetera. Their bodies have never had to adjust to using protein foods for energy and they've also been much more active throughout their lives than most of us will ever be on a regular basis.

We recommend that you eat at least three main meals per day with frequent snacks in between, going no more than two hours or so without at least a handful of nuts or some lean protein. This will keep hunger at bay and keep your blood sugar and energy levels steady.

Cooking on the Paleo Diet

Many raw foods enthusiasts use some version of the Paleo Diet, although it takes a great deal of creativity and, in some cases, bravery. However, you should eat as much of your fruits, veggies, nuts and seeds in a raw state as possible. Cooking changes the chemical structure of all foods, making them less digestible and even less tasty. It also destroys many of the vitamins that the foods contain. Be sure to eat plenty of raw fruits and veggies in particular.

When it is time to cook, there are best practices for cooking your food on the Paleo Diet. Grilling, steaming, roasting, baking and broiling enhance food's flavor, preserve the most nutrients and don't require added oils. Always opt for one of these methods. Stir-frying is also acceptable, but less often, as you will need to add oil to most dishes. When you do, choose extra virgin olive oil for sautéing or stir-frying and canola oil for baking. Deep-frying is never okay.

Did you know? A Note About Brown-Bagging: A frequent complaint among new Paleo followers is that it's hard to find lunch ideas for work when you can't have sandwiches made with bread or traditional wraps. The easiest solution is salads that include plenty of lean protein, hearty soups or just a selection of leftover meat (such as cold chicken legs) and some fruits and veggies. One thing that will help a great deal is to double up on dinner recipes so that you have planned leftovers, or to cook batches of things like chicken breasts on the weekend so you have them handy throughout the week.

When cooking vegetables, learn to enjoy them crisp – you'll get more fiber and more nutrients and feel more satisfied by the crunch and texture of al dente veggies.

Soups and stews are a real boon to the Paleo Diet. You can follow specific recipes or just toss in whatever you have handy or have a taste for eating. They're great for freezing extra servings and are easy to take to work and reheat for lunch.

Creating a Meal Plan

Even if you typically plan meals on the fly, you should definitely try doing some menu planning each week. It's important that you have what you need on hand so that you're able to follow the diet with each meal and snack, rather than setting yourself up to be tempted by the vending machine or drive-thru.

Use the foods list and supermarket guide as a starting place, then choose some of the recipes in the included Paleo Diet Solution Cookbook or from one of the many Paleo recipe sites online to create your meal plan. Whenever possible, cook ahead on the weekends, prepare cut fruits and veggies for lunches and snacks and make several servings of salad. This will help you to avoid having to spend a great deal of time prepping and cooking each day and make it easier for you to make smart choices. Keep a stash of non-perishable snacks such as nuts, dried fruits and seeds at work so that you always have a Paleo-friendly snack handy to ward off cravings and keep your energy high.

What You'll Be Eating

We'll go into much greater detail on specific foods on the foods list, but here is an overview of what you're allowed to eat on your Paleo Diet.

Firstly, know that all grains, processed foods, sugar and alcohol are out. These are not to be eaten at all, even in moderation. Don't worry, after a few weeks, you won't miss them.

PROTEINS

Your animal proteins will come from either livestock animals or game animals. Your livestock meats will come from lean beef, pork and lamb that is grass fed and organic. You can enjoy any cut you like at least some of the time. If you're in the mood for a less-lean cut, simply trim as much fat as possible, but make the majority of cuts the leaner ones, such as loins and filets. Bacon is acceptable as a flavoring or very occasionally as a dish, but only the lean parts – fat should be trimmed before cooking.

Game meats and game birds, such as venison, buffalo, ostrich, pheasant, quail and other smaller game are very good choices and are more widely available today than ever before. They are typically far lower in saturated fats than many livestock animals and you may enjoy trying many new flavors of meat.

Poultry such as chicken, turkey, duck, goose and Cornish hens should be organic, free-range, vegetarian-fed animals.

Eggs are an excellent source of protein on the Paleo diet, as long as they are from organic, free-range birds.

Seafood such as fish, shrimp, crab, clams, oysters and lobster is another excellent source of protein. You should get as many servings as possible from cold-water fish such as cod, salmon and haddock to get the maximum Omega 3 content.

FRUITS AND VEGETABLES

When it comes to fruits and vegetables, the sky is almost the limit. Try to stick to low-glycemic varieties for the majority of your meals and snacks. However, because you're cutting out grains and processed foods, you are still free to enjoy the high-glycemic varieties of produce for some of your snacks and meals. Here are some examples of fruits and vegetables based on their glycemic index:

Lower-Glycemic Fruits and Vegetables: Cantaloupe, rhubarb, apples, apricots, bananas, grapefruit, lemons and limes, oranges, plums, strawberries, asparagus, broccoli, cabbage, cauliflower, celery, cucumber, endive lettuce, radishes, mustard greens, spinach, Swiss chard, watercress.

Higher-Glycemic Fruits and Vegetables: Watermelon, blueberries, figs, grapes, mangoes, pears, pineapple, Brussels sprouts, chives, dandelion leaves, kale, leeks, okra, onions, parsley, peppers, artichokes, carrots.

You should buy organic whenever possible (or better yet, grow at least some of them), but in our section on eating Paleo on a budget and in our shopping guide, we'll show you how to prioritize your organics if money or availability is an issue.

Frozen fruits and veggies are acceptable, but try to keep them at a minimum. Canned vegetables and fruits should not be eaten – they contain too much salt and are overcooked, which means they have less fiber and fewer nutrients.

NUTS, SEEDS AND OILS

The rest of your foods will be made up of nuts, seeds and oils. For nuts, you'll eat tree nuts, such as walnuts, pecans and almonds (as opposed to peanuts, which are actually a legume and off-limits). These should be eaten raw whenever possible, or at least roasted without sugar, salt or added oil. Avocadoes are another delicious and nutritious choice. Seeds such as sunflower seeds, pumpkin seeds and sesame seeds are a great snack or baking ingredient.

You should use extra virgin olive oil for dressings and for sautéing foods. For the best flavor, use the lighter versions for eating raw and the less-costly regular versions for cooking. Since most baked goods such as cookies and bars don't taste too great made with olive oil, you can use canola oil for baking.

These are your basic guidelines and a rundown of the foods you'll be eating. We'll go into more detail throughout the rest of this book, but this lets you know what's involved and what to expect from the Paleo Diet.

CHAPTER 11

Foods Not Allowed on the Paleo Diet

W e give you a list of the allowed foods on the Paleo Diet on our Paleo Foods List in the Paleo Diet Solution Shopping Guide, but for clarity, here is a list of foods that are not allowed, or are allowed only occasionally or in very small amounts.

Dairy Foods

- All foods made with any dairy products
- Butter
- Cheese
- Nonfat dairy creamer
- Skim milk
- Dairy spreads
- Powdered Milk
- Frozen yogurt
- Ice Milk
- Low-fat Milk
- Ice cream
- Whole Milk
- Yogurt

Cereal Grains

- Barley (barley soup, barley bread and all processed foods made with barley)
- Corn (corn on the cob, corn tortillas, corn chips, cornstarch, corn syrup)
- Millet
- Oats (steel-cut oats, rolled oats and all processed foods made with oats)
- Rice (brown rice, white rice, top ramen, rice noodles, basmati rice, rice cakes, rice flour and all processed foods made with rice)
- Rye (rye bread, rye crackers and all processed foods made with rye)
- Sorghum
- Wheat (bread, rolls, muffins, noodles, crackers, cookies, doughnuts, pancakes, waffles, pasta, spaghetti, lasagna, wheat tortillas, pizza, pita bread, flat bread and all processed foods made with wheat or wheat flour)

Cereal Grain-like Seeds

- Amaranth
- Buckwheat
- Quinoa

Legumes

- All beans (adzuki beans, black beans, broad beans, fava beans, field beans, garbanzo beans, horse beans, kidney beans, lima beans, mung beans, navy beans, pinto beans, red beans, string beans, white beans)
- Black-eyed peas
- Chickpeas
- Peanuts
- Lentils
- Snow peas
- Peas
- Sugar snap peas
- Peanut butter
- Miso
- Soybeans and all soybean products, including tofu

Starchy Vegetables

- Cassava root
- Yams
- Tapioca
- Manioc
- Potatoes and all potato products (French fries, potato chips…)

High-Salt Foods

- Processed Meats
- Pork rinds
- Salami
- Deli Meats
- Kielbasa or smoked sausage
- Hot Dogs
- Ketchup
- Pickled foods
- Olives
- Salted nuts
- Salted spices
- Sausages
- Smoked, dried and salted fish / meat
- Virtually all canned meats or fish

Fatty Meats

- Bacon (use lean portions sparingly for seasoning and cooking)
- Fatty beef roasts
- Beef ribs
- Fatty ground beef
- T-bone steaks
- Chicken and turkey legs

- Chicken and turkey skin
- Chicken and turkey thighs and wings
- Fatty pork chops
- Fatty pork roasts
- Pork ribs
- Pork sausage
- Lamb chops
- Lamb roasts
- Leg of lamb

CHAPTER 12

Transitioning to the Paleo Lifestyle

Any healthy lifestyle change is more likely to be a success if you do a little planning. Knowing what to expect and positioning yourself for a change in habits, lifestyle and choices will make the transition easier, more pleasant, quicker and more likely to stick. Here are some things that will help you before you get started on the Paleo Diet and during your first few weeks of eating like your ancestors.

Before You Start Your Diet

We're all for enthusiasm and excitement about starting your Paleo lifestyle, but it's a good idea to give yourself a week or two to get ready for the transition. The Paleo Diet requires you to make some real changes in your eating and buying and meal-planning habits. You'd do well to lay the groundwork before you begin. Here are some things you should do before your first day on the diet.

Get Rid of the Forbidden Stuff

First, stop buying off-limits foods immediately. That means no processed foods, no sugar, no coffee, no flour or products made with flour, such as bread, crackers, cookies, cakes, gravy mixes, muffins, bagels, tortillas, etc.

Then you need to eat up or get rid of what you already have in the house. If you're too gung-ho to eat what's in your pantry or fridge, then by all means get rid of it instead. We're not suggesting your throw these foods away – that would be irresponsible. Here are some ideas for getting the foods out of your house:

- Donate unopened foods to a local shelter or food bank.

- Pass food boxes on to family members, friends and neighbors.

- Take canned goods to your grocery store's food donation bin or give them to the mailman if they're having their food drive.

- Take snack foods, canned fruits, unopened cereal or juices to a local day care center.

- Give unwanted items to your church or community group.

The important thing is to make sure that all of the forbidden foods are out of your house at least a couple of days before you start your diet.

> *Did you know?* *For Paleos Living With Non-Paleos: If you live with roommates or family members who will not be starting the Paleo Diet with you, try to keep the forbidden foods in one cupboard, one section of the fridge or one area of the pantry. If possible, make these the areas that are above or below eye level, so that they aren't staring you in the face at all times.*

Don't forget to get rid of any candy, soda, chips or other off-limit foods at work. Give your stash to co-workers or take them to a friend.

Find New Food Sources

We'll go into more detail shortly about how to shop on the Paleo Diet. It's possible to eat a Paleo Diet by shopping at your favorite grocery store, but some foods, such as nut flours, wild game or organic produce are easier to find elsewhere. Once you've read the shopping guidelines, do some research to decide where and how you'll be getting your groceries. There are great sources available, both online and locally – find them before you get started. If you're going to be using online purveyors, you'll need to order in time to have those supplies on hand for your first week.

Did you know? A Note to The Highly Caffeinated. If you are seriously dependent on coffee, black tea, colas or iced tea, read our section on caffeine and start taking the recommended steps to cutting out caffeine, or at least cutting way back. It's best to start this process at least a week before you start your diet.

Spread the Word

Unless you're the sole inhabitant of a backwoods cabin or a deserted island, you're going to need to prepare the people around you for your lifestyle change. This will enable them to support you and will help you avoid unintended sabotage or temptation from friends who may not take you seriously, or who just may be unaware that you're making a lifestyle change.

Let your friends, relatives and co-workers know that you're going on the Paleo Diet and give them an idea of what that means without going over more details than they'd like to hear. Let them know that you love their chocolate cake but prefer they don't bring one to your next dinner party, or that you may not be able to join them for lunch at the deli.

It's especially important to let roommates and the other members of your household know what you're doing and why. They don't have to join you or even agree with you, but they should be supportive and respectful. If you talk to them beforehand and let them know that you're excited about making a healthy change to your lifestyle, they'll be much more likely (and able) to encourage and help you.

During the First Few Weeks

Any diet comes with an adjustment period. The Paleo Diet is very different from the diet you've probably been eating most of your life. Give your mind and your body time to make the adjustment.

During the first couple of weeks, you may notice that your energy is flagging. You may want to jot a note down on your calendar to track any patterns. If you see that you tend to start dragging at 3pm, when you used to have your cola or candy bar, you may need to plan for a 3pm snack. If you're really feeling lethargic or if you get lightheaded when you exercise, add some high-glycemic carbs to your pre-workout meal or cut back temporarily on the length or intensity of your workouts. This phase will pass in just a couple of weeks.

Take care to avoid your weak spots or times when you used to be most likely to have sweets, coffee or alcohol. Skip happy hour with your office buddies, catch up on office news somewhere other than at the vending machine or cafeteria, or go for a walk instead of plopping in front of the TV after dinner.

By preparing yourself for your first few weeks on the Paleo Diet, you will greatly reduce the adjustment time and greatly increase your chances of successfully sticking to the diet.

CHAPTER 13

Sourcing and Shopping for Food

In the Paleo Diet Solution Shopping Guide at the back of the book, you'll find a handy shopping list and a section-by-section guide to shopping for groceries at your local supermarket. While you can get most of your groceries at your local supermarket, some things may be unavailable or of lesser quality at the local grocery store. Here we discuss some other good sources for getting the foods you'll be eating on the Paleo Diet.

Local Farms

With the resurgence of specialized and small family farms, even the most urban areas have small, organic farms nearby. Of particular interest to those on a Paleo Diet are what are known as CSA (Community Sustained Agriculture) Farms. These farms allow you to purchase a membership at very low cost, which allows you to purchase a week's or a month's worth of organic meats, eggs or produce as they become available. Many of these CSA farms also offer such foods as buffalo, ostrich or game birds.

Other local farms are equally good resources. Many let you pick your own fruits, veggies and berries, or have a farm stand either on their property or at local farmer's markets. Farmer's markets are also a good source of organic, local honey, eggs and herbs.

Health Food and Whole Foods Stores

If your grocery store has an extensive organic or health food section, you may be able to get everything you need there. However, whole foods markets and health food stores may be a better bet for things like bulk foods, raw nuts, nut butters, nut flours, seeds and oils.

Because of the competition from bigger, mainstream markets, health food stores and whole food groceries are often competitively priced and many offer sales and coupons that make them very affordable.

Online Resources

The Internet is a great resource for many foods that may not be available to you locally.

Wild game and meats like bison or venison can be especially hard to find, but the popularity of the Paleo Diet has brought about a surge of providers who sell their products online. You can order dressed game birds, venison stew meat and steaks and just about anything else you can think of from small producers all over the country. Just be sure to do your research to make sure they are responsible producers and don't assume that all providers raise their stock organically. If it isn't stated upfront, ask. These sources can be a bit expensive, but if you get the majority of your foods locally, you can take some of that money you were spending on fast food and sugary treats and use it to broaden your online horizons.

CHAPTER 14

Paleo Economy: Going Paleo on a Budget

In today's economy, most of us are on a budget, especially when it comes to food shopping. While some people have more to spend each week on food than others, if you're on a tight budget, there are some things you can do to help you follow the Paleo Diet without having to scrimp in other areas. The Paleo Diet has a somewhat misguided reputation as being expensive to follow, but this isn't true at all. As with all food shopping, you can make your grocery bill as high as you want or as low as you need it to be by making the choices that are best for your needs and your finances.

Prioritize Your Organics

The only absolute rule when it comes to buying organic is when you're shopping for meats and eggs. These must be organic, grass fed and free-range animals and eggs from vegetarian-fed, free-range birds.

You can buy whatever seafood is freshest or most attractive to you. Fresh is best, frozen is fine, but organic is not necessary.

When it comes to fruits and vegetables, organic is best, but if you can't afford to buy all organic produce, if some items aren't available or if you need something that's out of season, you can prioritize your organic choices. Fruits that are thick skinned and will be peeled before eating don't have to be organic. These include oranges, bananas, melons and any other fruit that will be peeled. Buy organic when purchasing apples, pears, peaches, grapes, cherries, berries and other fruits that won't be peeled. Even if you plan to peel your apples, they are thin-skinned and harmful chemicals can seep through that thin peel, so always go with the organic variety.

Buy in Bulk

After a few weeks or a month on the Paleo Diet, you'll be able to identify certain foods that you use a lot, such as chicken breasts, turkey legs, raw almonds or nut flours. Once you know you'll be using these foods a lot, buy in bulk whenever you can. Large packages and foods sold loosely in bins are often available (even in organic varieties), and these are usually much less costly per pound. There are wholesale butchers who can give you a special deal on larger orders of organic meats, too.

Cook in Bulk

To save both time and money, cook ahead in batches whenever you can. Make six chicken breasts or roast two birds at once and freeze or refrigerate the rest for lunches or for dinners on especially hectic evenings. You'll save money by avoiding impulse spending and even by conserving electricity. This is also a great way to take advantage of an especially good sale without risking the food spoiling before you can use it.

Use Everything!

By getting creative about using up everything you buy, you can save a surprising amount of money. For instance, whole chickens cost much less per pound than cut up chicken parts. Multiple meals can be squeezed from one bird:

- Cut the wings and legs off for roasting one meal.

- Simmer the rest of the bird with some water, herbs and carrot/celery tops.

- Remove all of the meat.

- Set aside some of the meat for salads and/or a casserole – you'll easily get enough for one meal.

- Use the remaining meat by returning it to the soup, which you can use as a base for several different soup meals.

Create vegetable stock for soups and stews by simmering the cuttings from carrots, celery, beets, turnips, greens and other veggies. Throw in a little sea salt and some herbs and you'll have several cups of stock that were virtually free.

Brown Bag Your Lunch

It's possible to stay on the Paleo Diet if you go out for lunch, but it's difficult and a lot more expensive than bringing your own lunch to work. By purposely cooking planned leftovers, making soups and stews and preparing plenty of high-protein salads, you can have a terrific and Paleo-friendly lunch for a fraction of the cost of eating out.

Get Coupons for Organic and Specialty Products

Coupons for organic foods and specialty health foods don't show up very often in the Sunday paper. However, they are available. Visit the websites of your local "healthy" supermarket, such as Earth Fare or Whole Foods – they often have coupons that have pretty high values. Sign up for any newsletters, too, as they'll notify you of special sales and often have coupons attached just for subscribers. You can also email your favorite organic or health food brands to request coupons – most companies have them available, even if they don't distribute them to the newspapers. Many of these companies also have special deals for customers who "Like" their Facebook pages.

Grow Your Own

If you're fortunate enough to have the time and space for a large kitchen garden, good for you! You'll save a ton of money this way and be assured of organic products at the peak of freshness. However, don't let the lack of acreage or lots of free time discourage you. Even if all you can do is plant a few containers of tomatoes, peppers and other veggies, you'll save a great deal.

Growing your own herbs is another great way to save a significant amount of money. The Paleo Diet relies on herbs fairly heavily. Fresh herbs are better than dried, but they can get pretty expensive. Luckily, you can grow many of them for actual pennies, and right in your kitchen windowsill, on your fire escape or in your flower beds. Thyme, chives, rosemary, parsley, oregano, sage, mint and dill are a few of the ones most often seen in meat and seafood recipes, so they're a good place to start, but you can add in your own favorites, too.

Try CSA Farms

We talked about CSA Farms earlier, and they're a great way to get the freshest produce, eggs and meat and save a ton of money at the same time. Prices are usually based on a whole growing season (anywhere from six to twelve months depending on where you live) and are quoted per person. Some farms just sell produce, while others sell only orchard and vine fruits and still others sell only meats or one type of meat.

Produce is easiest to find from CSA farms and you'll reap tremendous savings. For as little as $400 or so per season for a family of four, you'll be allowed to pick up a week's worth of whatever has been harvested that week.

Meat is also usually significantly cheaper from CSA farms, even compared to non-organic meats at your local supermarket. Price is usually per pound for a quarter, side or whole animal, regardless of what cuts of meat are included. Steaks cost the same as ground beef and vice versa. When you crunch the numbers, $4-7 a pound (fairly typical price range) for a larger order is a great deal.

Go To Sea

No, you don't need to catch your own fish, although that's certainly a great way to spend a day outdoors and save money at the same time. However, if organic meats are difficult for you to afford, focus the majority of your meals on seafood proteins. The price per pound may not be much less, but you'll need less of it to make a meal. A pound of shrimp goes much farther than a pound of steak.

Buy Turkey

Turkey is the ramen noodle of animal protein. Sometimes less than a dollar per pound, it's a true bargain and you can cook once and have enough meat for ten, twenty or more meals. If you have an extra freezer in your home or can borrow space in someone else's, buy several turkeys when they're pennies a pound during the holidays. The savings over chicken and other meats can run into hundreds of dollars per year.

Barter With a Gardening Friend

If you don't have space for a kitchen garden but you have a friend who does, ask if you can trade for fresh produce. You might be able to offer tutoring for their child, piano lessons, house painting, furniture refinishing, sewing or a multitude of other services in exchange for a basket of the freshest fruits and veggies every week or month.

Eat Seasonally as Much as Possible

Since there were no supermarkets or trucking companies in the Stone Age, people ate fruits and vegetables at the peak of freshness and nutrition, often immediately after picking. By eating seasonally whenever possible, you'll pay much less per pound for your produce. Apples and pears are cheaper by as much as a dollar per pound in the fall and asparagus, peaches, cherries and grapes cost much less in spring and summer.

You'll be able to find plenty of ways to cut the cost of shopping for your Paleo foods. Use your creativity, be open to trying new foods and new ways to prepare cheaper items, and always keep your eyes open for a good bargain.

CHAPTER 15

A Day in the Life of the Modern Caveperson

Each person is an individual, with different appetites, schedules, routines and habits. However, you'll benefit from having a guideline on how to spread out both your nutrition and your cooking/prep time on the Paleo Diet. This is just a guideline for you to use to get started; you'll likely tweak this as you go through your first few weeks on the diet.

Early Morning/Breakfast

Eat as early as possible after you awaken, especially during your first few weeks. After a few weeks, your body will begin utilizing protein better for energy. If you keep your evening meals protein heavy and carb light, you'll awaken with more energy in the morning, without having to reach for coffee or carbs to get going.

In the first few weeks, your breakfast should be a good, solid serving of protein such as meat or eggs, coupled with veggies and low-glycemic fruits. Scrambles and omelets are a good choice if you have time. If you have little time for cooking in the morning, smoothies, cold leftover meats and raw fruit are good.

Morning Snack

Your morning snack should be no later than two hours after breakfast, to keep your energy levels and blood sugar steady. Combine a serving of protein and a serving of carbs.

Lunch

Lunch should be no later than two hours after your morning snack. You should get a good helping of proteins here, such as a meat soup or stew, cold leftover chicken or a salad with chicken breast or leftover roast beef or shrimp. Accompany this with high-fiber carbs for extra fullness, such as a salad, apples and a handful of nuts.

Afternoon Snack

Eat an afternoon snack no later than two hours after lunch. You may find that this is when you need carbs the most, as you're likely used to an afternoon latte or candy bar. Eat a high-glycemic fruit such as grapes, a banana or some berries. Dried fruits are also a good choice here. Add some nuts or a bit of protein for fullness.

Dinner

Your evening meals should focus primarily on protein. Most people require less energy during the evening; unless you work out after dinner, go easy on the carbs. Choose low-glycemic veggies as your sides or just have the meat or seafood.

Dessert or Evening Snack

You're free to choose between a sweet treat or just a little more food, whatever you like. Fruit, fruit ices and any of the Paleo-friendly dessert recipes in the included Paleo Diet Solution Cookbook will all satisfy a sweet tooth. If you just need a bite to eat, focus more on protein.

Cooking and Prep

If at all possible, try to prepare tomorrow's lunch and snacks while you're cooking tonight's dinner. This will save you time, ensure that you have Paleo-friendly meals ready to go and keep you from adding chaos to your mornings. Just pack up leftovers from dinner, add some fruits, nuts and other snacks and you're all set.

Did you know? *Water, Water Everywhere: It's essential for all of us to get plenty of water each day, but on the Paleo Diet, water is pretty much all you get. Look into purchasing reusable water bottles or bottles with filters built right in. You'll save money on buying bottled water every week. Extra Tip: Freeze your water overnight – it'll be wonderfully cold all day and keep your lunch refrigerated, too.*

CHAPTER 16

The Paleo Diet and Working Out

Regular strength-training and cardio exercise is important on any diet and the Paleo Diet is no exception. If you already work out regularly, you may need to make some adjustments. If you haven't been on a workout program, now is a good time to start, but you'll want to take it easy during the first few weeks.

For Those Already Working Out Regularly

We discussed nutrition and exercise in our section on the Paleo Diet for Athletes, but even if you're not an athlete, you may need to scale back a bit on your workouts the first few weeks of your Paleo Diet.

You are likely going to be reducing your overall carb intake somewhat, unless you were already on a high-protein, low-carb diet. It may take your body a few weeks to adjust to having mostly protein to work with for quick or sustained energy.

You'll feel this less when it comes to strength-training, although you may find that shorter workouts are better, just for a few weeks. After those initial weeks, you'll notice a dramatic increase in strength, energy and endurance and you can ramp your workouts back up again.

If your workouts include sustained or intense cardio training or any kind of high-intensity interval training, you may want to cut back the intensity level or length of your workouts. Intervals may be better set aside for the first few weeks.

Feel free to try your normal workout the first few days. You may find that you notice no difference. In that case, carry on as usual.

If you feel slightly dizzy or lightheaded during your workout, rest and have a snack, then start eating a bit of protein and some carbs 15-30 minutes prior to your workouts.

For Those Just Starting a Workout Program

Even though we tend to get excited and enthusiastic about changing our lifestyles and our bodies, it's always best to start slowly when embarking on a workout program, especially if you've been sedentary for some time, are significantly overweight or have any health issues, such as diabetes, heart problems or back/neck trouble.

Always seek your doctor's advice before starting a workout program and ask if there are any limitations to what you should do.

You need both resistance training (for building and reshaping muscle, speeding metabolism and strengthening bones) and cardio exercise (for calorie burning and cardiovascular health) to change and maintain your body. You can exercise every day or every other day, but you should get 30 minutes of exercise at least three times a week as a minimum.

You don't have to join a gym or buy expensive equipment to get started. A small set of dumbbells and some inexpensive resistance bands are great for strength training. Push-ups, pull-ups, squats and lunges are still some of the best strength moves around and you don't have to buy a thing. Choose a few moves for each body part, use core and combination moves (such as weighted lunges) to get the most benefit in the least time, and gradually build up your sets and reps.

As you gain strength and experience, you can amp it up by increasing weight, using slow-lifting techniques or integrating interval training into your workouts.

Walking, swimming, cycling and dancing are all great ways to get your cardio and they're excellent choices for the beginner, because chances for injury are lower than with some other forms of exercise. Buy decent shoes for your sport, but go easy on the workout clothing and gadgets unless you can easily afford them or they really aid your motivation.

Start slowly, always warm up for at least five minutes prior to and cool down for at least five minutes after every workout. Measure your progress in reps, weight, blocks walked or minutes spent dancing. No matter how you choose to measure your progress and increase your intensity, be sure to give yourself credit for every goal met.

SECTION THREE

Living With Your Inner Caveman

CHAPTER 17

What about Eating Out?

Eating out is a challenge when you're on a diet or special eating plan, but the Paleo Diet is less troublesome than most. It's certainly easier to prepare your own food when you're on the Paleo Diet, but there's no reason why you shouldn't enjoy restaurant meals, too. Just follow these simple guidelines and you'll have little trouble enjoying a nice meal with friends and family.

If at All Possible, Eat at Organic Restaurants

The popularity of raw and organic eating has made organic foods much more available in many restaurants and organic restaurants have popped up in most urban areas. If you have a choice, frequent these establishments, which generally offer only organic meats and seafood and locally grown, in-season produce.

When Organic Isn't Available, Compromise

If you can't go to an organic restaurant, you may still have organic options at another favorite eatery. If organic meats aren't on the menu, go for the seafood instead, as organic seafood is less crucial than organic meats.

If all else fails, have a chicken leg or two before you go out and order a vegetarian entrée.

Try to Keep the No-No's Away From the Table

Obviously, you'll have to consider your dining companions, but if possible, ask the server not to bring bread, butter, crackers or breadsticks to the table.

Advise your server that you're on a gluten-free, dairy-free diet – they may have some suggestions for you. If not, they'll at least be able to advise the cook, who should be prepared with substitutions for allergic guests.

Order your entrees without sauces, gravies or dressings and ask for vinaigrette or oil and vinegar if you're having a salad. Make sure they leave off the croutons, too.

If your entrée comes with a choice of potato or pasta, request steamed veggies or an extra helping of salad instead. Most restaurants are prepared for this and happy to accommodate you.

Maybe You Can't Have Your Cake and Eat It Too

Unless your restaurant has a fruit plate, you may be out of luck when it comes to dessert. Instead of feeling deprived, focus on enjoying your entrée and the good company.

If you only eat out very occasionally and you have pretty good willpower, share a forbidden dessert with one of your companions. A couple of bites of cake or ice cream won't kill you as long as it's a very rare thing. Don't beat yourself up about it, either.

CHAPTER 18

Where's My Caffeine? Help for the Really Addicted

One of the real sticking points for some people is the lack of caffeine on the Paleo Diet. This can even be a deal-breaker for some. If you're seriously dependent on your coffee, cola and sweet tea to get you through the day, we'll be honest: this part will be tough. However, it is do-able.

If at all possible, start weaning yourself from your caffeine about two weeks before you start your diet.

If you're a coffee drinker, cut down from four to two cups, only drink coffee in the morning, or gradually lessen the strength of your coffee. You can mix it with water, switch from espresso to regular coffee, or blend decaf with regular grounds. If you use milk or sugar, gradually start cutting back on those, too, since they're both off-limits.

Try switching from coffee to black tea to get your caffeine fix. Then move on to substituting green or herbal tea. Try to refrain from sweetening it with anything other than honey.

Sodas are out on the Paleo Diet, so start cutting back and finding substitutions. Go from cola to clear sodas and from clear sodas to water, or just quit cold turkey if you can. In a pinch, try iced green tea or water with some fruit juice or fruit slices.

If you are a serious addict and simply cannot give up the coffee, at least try to gradually cut out the milk and sugar. Non-dairy creamer is also unacceptable, so skip it. If you can get yourself to drink your coffee black and keep it at a bare minimum, you can get away with it. It's better than skipping the Paleo Diet altogether.

CHAPTER 19

Vitamin Supplements on the Paleo Diet

A well-rounded Paleo Diet provides plenty of most vitamins and minerals, but there are a few that you may   need to get from a supplement. Bear in mind that the increased intake of plant fibers and antioxidants means that you're getting more antioxidants through your food and at the same time not eating oxidative foods, which compete with vitamins for absorption, so you can get less than the RDA of many vitamins and minerals.

Vitamin D

Vitamin D is the most common nutrient that people bring up when debating the healthiness of the Paleo Diet. While it is true that we get most of our Vitamin D from dairy foods, you will get small amounts in other foods, especially oily fish such as mackerel and sardines. However, if you're not that crazy about oily fish and you can't get at least 30 minutes of sunlight every day, you may want to take a Vitamin D supplement. Between 1,000 and 4,000 IU of vitamin D3 in gel caps seems to be the ideal.

Iron

If you don't really care for beef or leafy greens, you may want to add an iron supplement. Check with your doctor before you do – excess iron can lead to constipation, digestive disorders and other issues.

Omega 3 or Fish Oil

If seafood isn't your thing, you may want to add a fish oil supplement to your diet. You'll get Omega 3s in organic, grass fed meats, but there's almost no chance of too much of a good thing when it comes to Omega 3.

Probiotics

Probiotics are often found today in commercially available yogurts and milk, but you won't get them that way on the Paleo Diet. Your Paleo Diet is rich in antioxidants, but if you are under a good deal of stress or are prone to digestive disorders, we recommend a high potency and high quality probiotic including multiple strains of lactobacillus and bifido-bacterium. Several companies are offering pro-biotic supplements specially formulated for those on the Paleo Diet. You can find these supplements by doing a quick search online.

THE **PALEO** DIET SOLUTION

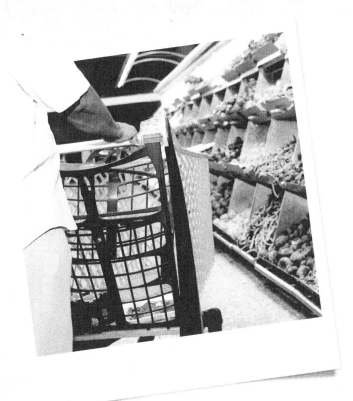

SHOPPING
GUIDE

ROCKRIDGE
UNIVERSITY PRESS

Here is an extensive list of the foods allowed on the Paleo Diet. You may want to print several copies so that you can take them to the store with you or use them to plan meals. Immediately following is our section-by-section Supermarket Shopping Guide.

Meats and Seafood

Lean Beef (trimmed of visible fat)

- Flank Steak
- Top Sirloin Steak
- Extra Lean hamburger (7% fat or less)
- London broil
- Lean veal
- Chuck Steak
- Any other lean cut

Lean Pork (trimmed of visible fat)

- Pork loin
- Pork Chops
- Any other lean cut

Lean poultry (white meat, skin removed)

- Chicken breast
- Turkey breast
- Game hen breasts

Eggs

- Whole eggs (Although many diets recommend only eating the whites, whole eggs are recommended for the Paleo diet. You can have eggs from chickens, ducks or geese. Do not buy egg substitutes.)

Rabbit meat (any cut)

Goat meat (any cut)

Organ meats

- Beef, lamb, pork, chicken livers and kidneys
- Chicken or turkey gizzards and hearts
- Beef, pork and lamb tongues
- Beef, lamb and pork marrow
- Beef, lamb and pork sweetbreads

Game meat (A-Z)

- Alligator
- Bear
- Bison (buffalo)
- Caribou
- Elk
- Emu
- Goose
- Kangaroo
- Muscovy duck
- New Zealand Cervena deer
- Ostrich
- Pheasant
- Quail
- Rattlesnake
- Reindeer
- Squab
- Turtle
- Venison
- Wild boar
- Wild turkey

Fish

- Bass
- Bluefish
- Branzini (Mediterranean sea bass)
- Cod (Scrod is a young 2.5 lb. or less cod)
- Drum
- Eel
- Flatfish
- Grouper
- Haddock
- Halibut
- Herring
- Mackerel
- Monkfish
- Mullet
- Northern Pike
- Orange Roughy
- Perch
- Red snapper
- Rockfish
- Salmon (fillet, steak, patties, smoked)
- Sardines
- Scrod
- Shark
- Striped bass
- Sunfish
- Swordfish
- Tilapia
- Trout
- Tuna

- Turbot
- Walleye
- Any other commercially available fish

Shellfish

- Abalone
- Clams
- Crab
- Crayfish
- Lobster
- Mussels
- Oysters
- Scallops
- Shrimp

Fruits and Vegetables

Fruits

- Apple
- Apricot
- Avocado
- Banana
- Blackberries
- Boysenberries
- Blueberries
- Cantaloupe
- Carambola
- Cherries
- Cherimoya
- Cranberries
- Gooseberries

- Grapefruit
- Grapes
- Guava
- Honeydew melon
- Kiwi
- Lemon
- Lime
- Lychee
- Mango
- Nectarines
- Oranges
- Papaya
- Passion Fruit
- Pears
- Pineapple
- Peaches
- Persimmon
- Plums
- Pomegranate
- Raspberries
- Rhubarb
- Star Fruit
- Tangerine
- Watermelon
- All other fruits

Vegetables

- Artichoke
- Asparagus
- Beet Greens
- Beets
- Bell peppers
- Broccoli

- Brussels sprouts
- Cabbage
- Carrots
- Cauliflower
- Celery
- Collards
- Cucumber
- Dandelion
- Eggplant
- Endive
- Endive
- Green Onions
- Kale
- Kohlrabi
- Lettuce (except iceberg)
- Mushrooms
- Mustard Greens
- Onions
- Parsley
- Parsnip
- Peppers (all kinds)
- Pumpkin
- Purslane
- Radish
- Rutabaga
- Seaweed
- Spinach
- Squash (all kinds)
- Swiss chard
- Tomatillos
- Tomato
- Turnip greens
- Turnips
- Watercress
- Zucchini

Nuts, Seeds and Oils

- Almond butter
- Almonds
- Brazil Nuts
- Canola oil
- Cashews
- Chestnuts
- Flax seed
- Hazelnuts
- Macadamia Nuts
- Nut flour (almond or hazel-nut is recommended)
- Olive oil
- Pecans
- Pine Nuts
- Pistachios
- Pumpkin Seeds
- Sesame Butter or Tahini (pure and raw)
- Sesame Seeds
- Sunflower Seeds
- Walnuts

Beverages

- Green tea
- Herbal tea
- Moderate amounts of pure, organic fruit juice, no added sugar
- Water

Other

- Carob powder
- Dried fruits without added sugar
- Fresh and dried herbs
- Frozen fruits and fruit bars without added sugar
- Raw, organic honey
- Spices and seasonings

The Paleo Diet Supermarket Guide

The key to sticking to the Paleo Diet while doing your grocery shopping at a regular supermarket is to shop from the outer sections and almost skip the center aisles entirely.

Most supermarkets are set up with the meat, seafood, organic and produce aisles on the outer rings of the store and this is where you need to stay for the most part. We'll take a quick run through the typical departments to give you an idea of how to shop Paleo at your local supermarket.

THE PRODUCE DEPARTMENT

Almost half your food is going to come from this one department. Whether you're buying fruits or vegetables, you want to shop seasonally as much as possible, buying what is in season and at the peak of freshness and nutritional value.

Buy organic as much as possible, but if you need to prioritize your organic purchase, stick with organic for foods that you will be eating without peeling, such as grapes, summer squash, berries, pears, spinach and greens, tomatoes and so on. Foods you'll be peeling can be safely purchased and eaten if you need to pick and choose when to go organic.

To get the widest variety of nutrients and the most antioxidant content, think "rainbow." Foods that are darker in color, such as red, orange and yellow, are highest in antioxidants and many essential phytonutrients.

Choose dark green vegetables as well, especially spinach, kale, broccoli or collard greens.

Iceberg lettuce has little nutritional value, so opt for leaf lettuces and Romaine.

The only off-limits items are white potatoes and corn.

THE MEAT DEPARTMENT

Most supermarkets have an organic meat section, usually close to or within the butcher counter.

Read any packaging carefully to make sure your choice is organic, grass fed meat. Choose the leanest cuts for the most part, such as loins, filets and some roasts and steaks. Keep the fattier cuts to a minimum.

Organ meats can also be an excellent ingredient on your Paleo menu. If you're unfamiliar with them, try one new organ meat a week, such as tongue, kidneys, sweetbreads or liver, to see which ones you like. They're often much less expensive than other cuts.

THE SEAFOOD DEPARTMENT

Buy as much of your seafood fresh as you possibly can – the flavor and texture are usually better and generally the food hasn't traveled as far.

Be sure to read the signs, packaging, or ask the fishmonger if the seafood was previously frozen. If it has been frozen and thawed, you cannot safely refreeze it unless you cook it first. If thawed shrimp is on sale or much cheaper than frozen, by all means buy it – just quickly steam or boil it, pack in Ziploc bags and re-freeze for later. Otherwise, if fish or seafood has been thawed, only buy what you can eat in the next day or two.

No kind of fish or other seafood is off-limits, but do avoid "pre-seasoned" or prepared items. They often contain far too much salt and may also have MSG and other additives.

OTHER DEPARTMENTS

Skip the bakery, dairy, baked goods, chip, cookie, cereal and pasta aisles. There's nothing there for you!

Some other items you may need in other departments are:

Frozen Foods: Frozen vegetables are fine if fresh is out of season or unavailable, but buy plain, uncooked veggies, making sure no sauce or butter has been added. Fresh fruits can be nice to have on hand for baked desserts and smoothies. Frozen fish and seafood are fine in a pinch, as long as they haven't been prepared in any way. Check the organic/health food section first, as many stock frozen items and they're preferable to regular commercial products.

Canned, Bottled and Jarred Goods: Be sure to have plenty of olive oil, canola oil, vinegars, sea salt, spices and seasonings (especially salt substitutes). You may also find raw, organic honey and want mustard, organic broths and stocks, bottled water, some pure juices and some nut butters. As before, check the organic section first to see if the healthier versions of all of these are stocked there.

CONCLUSION

With these guidelines, you'll find it pretty easy to shop for your Paleo Diet without getting too tempted by forbidden foods or spending too much time wandering the aisles. The best advice: stick to the outer departments, dash into the middle to get tissue and dish detergent and get out as quickly as you can!

THE PALEO DIET SOLUTION

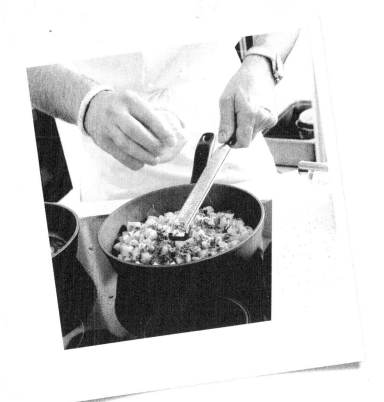

THE COOKBOOK

ROCKRIDGE UNIVERSITY PRESS

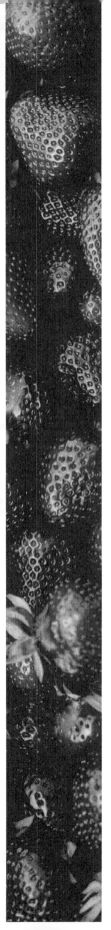

Stir-Fry Style Omelet

INGREDIENTS

- *3 eggs, beaten*
- *1 carrot sliced thin*
- *3 scallions cut to 1/2-inch slices*
- *1 cup broccoli florets*
- *1/2 cup cooked chicken*
- *Canola oil*
- *Salt*
- *Black pepper*

STEPS

Stir fry broccoli and carrot in a tablespoon of oil on medium heat until softened. Add cooked meat and stir fry until heated through. Add scallions and eggs, scramble. Add salt and pepper to taste. Serve.

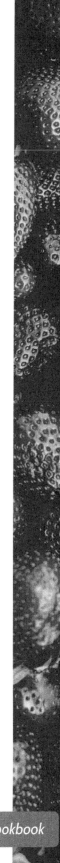

Garden of Eden Omelet

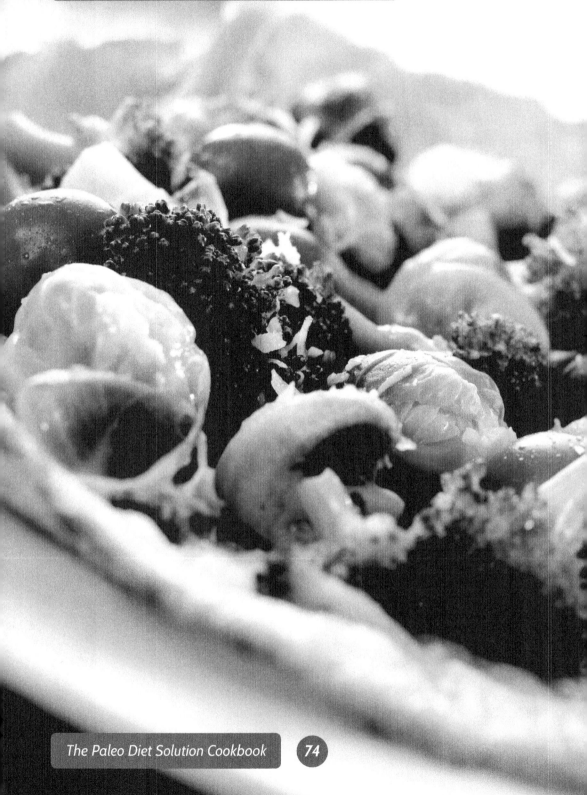

Garden of Eden Omelet

INGREDIENTS

- 1 cup of chopped fresh spinach
- 4 chopped green onions
- 1 clove of fresh chopped garlic
- 1/2 cup of sliced fresh mushrooms
- 4 eggs
- 1/4 cup V-8 juice
- Salt and pepper to taste
- 1 tbsp. olive oil

STEPS

Sauté chopped vegetables in hot olive oil. Beat eggs, V-8 juice and seasonings in bowl. Pour eggs over sautéed vegetables and cook until firm.

Turn omelet and cook other side until firm.

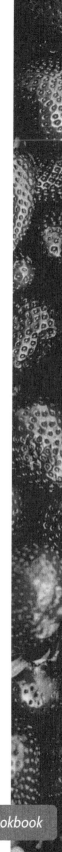

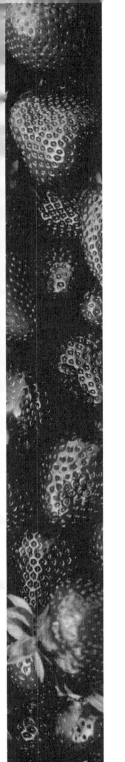

Nutty Spinach Quiche

INGREDIENTS

- Olive oil
- 1/4 cup raw sesame seeds
- 1 bunch kale
- 4 eggs
- 2 cloves minced garlic
- 1 cup chopped onions
- 1/2 cup chopped Canadian bacon
- 1 tsp brown mustard
- 1/4 tsp salt
- 1/4 tsp pepper

STEPS

Preheat oven to 375 degrees.

Grease a pie pan with olive oil and then coat pan with sesame seeds, shaking and turning pan to cover totally. Set aside.

Wash kale and cut out center ribs from leaves. Slice kale in ½-inch pieces. Place kale in a microwave safe bowl and microwave on high for one minute, or until just barely tender.

Add garlic and onion to bowl and microwave for one more minute. Squeeze out excess moisture by pressing with large spoon or spatula. Break eggs into a separate bowl and beat the eggs with a whisk until light and foamy. Add Canadian bacon, salt, pepper and mustard, mix well. Add kale mixture to eggs and pour into prepared pie pan and bake for 20-30 minutes until top looks dry and puffy. Serve hot or at room temperature.

Coconut Pancakes

INGREDIENTS

- 1/4 cup canola oil
- 1 dozen organic eggs, whipped
- 1 cup almond meal
- 1 cup unsweetened ground coconut meat
- 1/2 teaspoon salt
- 1 teaspoon cinnamon
- 1/2 teaspoon nutmeg
- Honey to taste

STEPS

Pour oil in an 11"x13" baking dish. Spread around and heat in 325-degree oven for 5 minutes.

In large mixing bowl, beat together all ingredients. Pour mixture into heated baking dish. Bake for 15-20 minutes until sides start to pull away and center is starting to crack. Serve with honey and garnish with fresh berries.

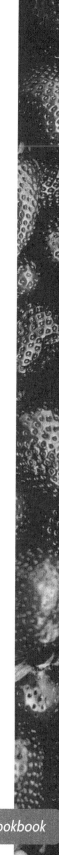

VERY BERRY PANCAKES

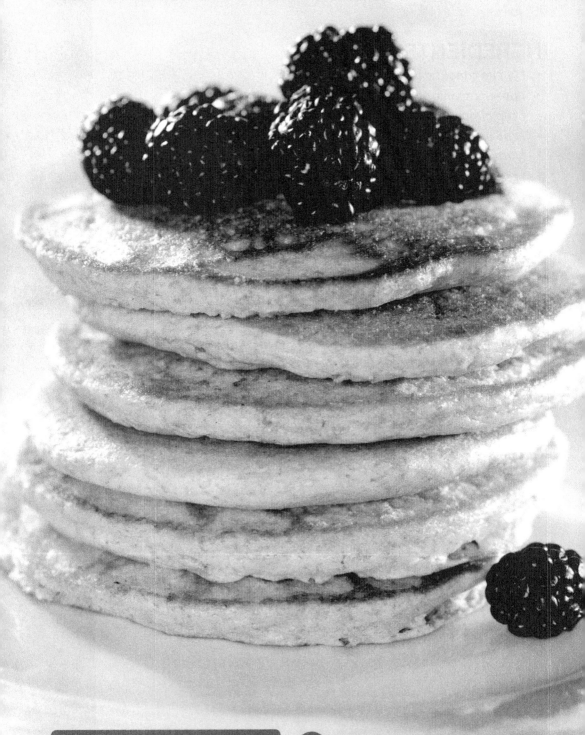

Very Berry Pancakes

INGREDIENTS

- 1 cup walnut meal
- 1/2 teaspoon sea salt
- 1 teaspoon baking powder
- 2 organic eggs
- 1 cup water
- 3 teaspoons walnut oil
- 1/2 cup chopped walnuts
- 1 cup blueberries (or other berries in season)

STEPS

Stir meal, salt and baking powder well. In separate bowl, whisk eggs and water. Stir eggs into meal and mix lightly. This will produce a thick batter. Fold in nuts and berries.

Cook each pancake in a little walnut or canola oil, turning once to cook both sides. Serves two.

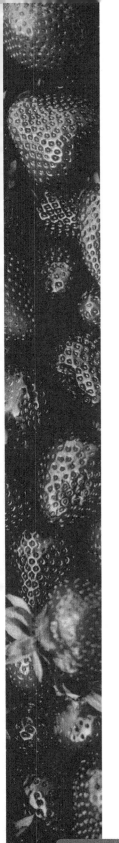

Nut Flour Muffins

INGREDIENTS

- 1 1/4 cups of nut flour (almond or walnut)
- 2 eggs
- 1 banana
- 1/8 cup of canola or walnut oil
- 1/2 cup fresh berries or chopped apple

STEPS

Preheat oven to 350 degrees and grease muffin pan.

Put everything except fruit in a food processor. Add fruit before spooning into greased muffin tins. Bake 12-15 minutes.

Fried Apples and Bacon

INGREDIENTS

- 4 Granny Smith apples peeled (or unpeeled) and chopped
- 1/2 lb. nitrate-free, maple-cured bacon, lean pieces only

STEPS

Fry bacon and drain on paper towel. Pour off all but 1 tablespoon drippings and fry apples in the hot bacon grease until soft. Crumble bacon, toss with apples and serve.

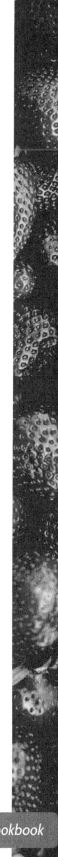

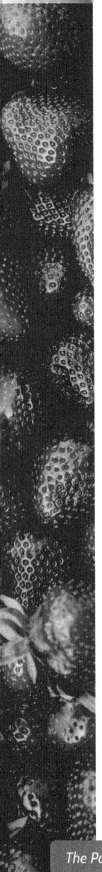

Creamy Hot Chocolate

INGREDIENTS

* 1 cup light coconut milk
* 1 tablespoon carob powder
* 1 teaspoon honey

STEPS

Combine coconut milk and carob powder. Blend with a wire whisk, heat on stovetop or in microwave. Add honey to taste.

Tuscan Eggs Cups

INGREDIENTS

- 6 large tomatoes
- 6 eggs
- 1/2 cup extra-virgin olive oil
- 1 garlic clove
- 1/2 cup fresh parsley
- 1/2 tsp sea salt
- 3/8 tsp freshly ground black pepper

STEPS

Add garlic, parsley, salt, pepper and olive oil to a food processor. Process until smooth.

Preheat oven to 400 degrees.

Core tomatoes and use a spoon to remove all the pulp and seeds.

Place the tomatoes in a lightly oiled 9" baking dish. Cover the bottom of each tomato with an equal amount of pesto sauce. Crack an egg into each tomato.

Season with additional salt and pepper to taste. Bake for approximately 20 minutes.

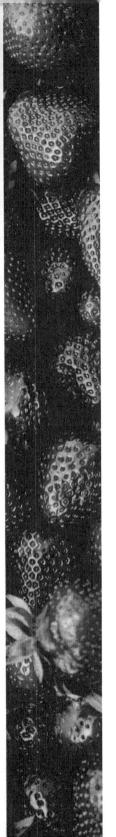

Portobello Egg Bake

INGREDIENTS
- 4 large Portobello mushrooms
- 4 eggs
- Cajun or Italian seasoning

STEPS

Break stems off mushrooms and use a spoon to scrape off the dark gills.

Crack an egg into each mushroom cap. Sprinkle with seasoning. Bake at 400 degrees for 15-30 minutes depending on how you like the yolk cooked: ~15 minutes for a runny yolk and up to 30 minutes for a firm yolk.

Sweet Potato Pancakes

INGREDIENTS

- 2 cups shredded sweet potatoes
- 1 apple shredded
- 1 small shallot chopped
- 2 eggs beaten
- 1 tsp cinnamon
- 1/2 tsp ground ginger
- 1 tsp lemon juice
- Canola oil for frying

STEPS

Mix all ingredients together well.

In a frying pan, heat coconut oil to medium heat.

Use about 1/4 cup of batter for each pancake.

Cook 3-5 minutes on each side until they are golden brown.

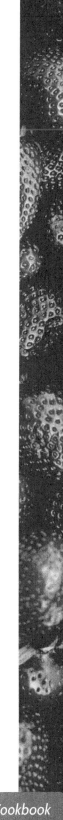

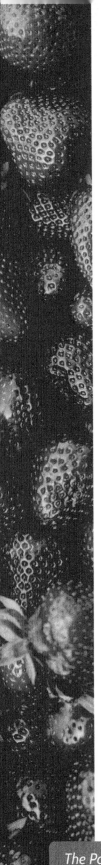

Baked Omelet Cups

INGREDIENTS

- 5 eggs
- 1/2 cup finely chopped cooked bacon
- 1/4 cup finely chopped onions
- 2 tablespoons chopped fresh parsley
- 1 teaspoon Cajun seasoning

STEPS

Whisk eggs and seasoning until light and fold in bacon, onions and parsley.

Spoon into oiled muffin tins.

Bake for 18-20 minutes until a knife comes out almost clean.

Rancho Luca Frittata

INGREDIENTS

- 1 bag fresh spinach
- 1 lb. cooked chicken breasts, boneless, cut into small pieces
- 1/4 cup extra virgin olive oil
- 3 garlic cloves, minced
- 1 red onion, chopped fine
- 1 red bell pepper, diced to 1/2 inch
- 1 green bell pepper, diced to 1/2 inch
- 1/4 cup chopped parsley
- 12 large eggs
- 1/2 teaspoon sea salt
- 1/2 teaspoon fresh ground black pepper

STEPS

Preheat oven to 375 degrees and coat the bottom and sides of a 9"x13" inch pan with oil.

Wash the spinach and place in a large pot. Cook over medium heat until just wilted. Set aside to cool. Sauté the onion in a large skillet over medium heat in one tablespoon oil until translucent. Add the garlic and bell pepper and continue cooking until the peppers are soft.

Break the eggs into a large bowl and whisk until light and frothy. Squeeze all the moisture from the spinach and add to eggs. Fold in the chicken, cooked peppers, salt and pepper.

Place in a 375-degree oven and bake for 1 hour, or until the top is brown and the center is firm.

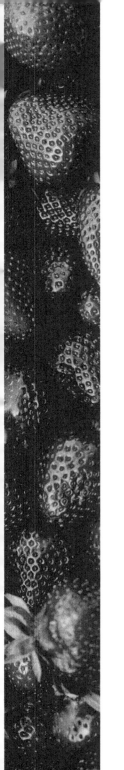

Turkey Breakfast Hash

INGREDIENTS

- 2 medium sweet potatoes, peeled and cut into 1/2-inch dice
- 1 green apple, cored and cut into 1/2-inch dice
- 1 teaspoon lemon juice
- 1 tablespoon olive oil
- 1 medium onion, chopped
- 3 cups diced, cooked, skinless turkey
- 1 tablespoon chopped fresh thyme
- 1 teaspoon ground sage
- 1/2 teaspoon salt
- Freshly ground pepper to taste

STEPS

In a medium saucepan, cover sweet potatoes with water and bring to a boil. Reduce heat to medium, cover and cook for 3 minutes. Add apple and cook until everything is just tender, but not mushy, 2 to 3 minutes longer. Drain.

Heat oil in a large nonstick skillet over medium-high heat. Add onion and cook, stirring often, until softened, 2 to 3 minutes. Add turkey, thyme, sage, salt and pepper; cook, stirring occasionally, until heated through, about 2 minutes. Add the reserved yam mixture to the pan; stir to mix. Press on the hash with a wide metal spatula; cook until the bottom is lightly browned, about 3 minutes. Turn the hash in sections and cook until the undersides are browned, about 3 minutes longer.

Summer Veggie Fritter

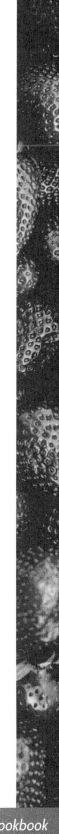

INGREDIENTS

- 2/3 cup sweet potato, grated
- 1/2 cup carrot, grated
- 1/2 cup red pepper, chopped fine
- 1/2 cup green peas
- 1/2 cup onion, chopped fine
- 1/2 cup almond meal
- 3 eggs
- Salt and pepper
- Coconut oil

STEPS

Combine all ingredients except for the coconut oil together in a mixing bowl.

Heat frying pan on medium heat and add some coconut oil.

Make patties with 1/3 cup batter. Cook on each side for 3-4 min, or until browned and cooked inside.

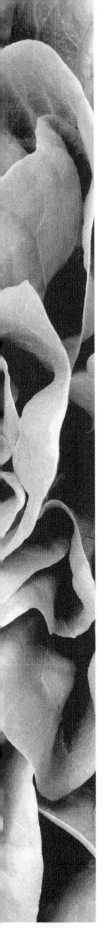

Lunch Recipes

Mushroom and Spring Greens Salad

INGREDIENTS

- 2 tablespoons fresh lemon juice
- 3 tablespoons extra virgin olive oil
- 1 minced garlic clove
- 2 tablespoons minced fresh parsley
- 1 teaspoon chopped fresh oregano or 1/4 teaspoon dry
- 1/4 teaspoon pepper
- 1 pound fresh mushrooms, very thinly sliced

STEPS

Combine the first six ingredients in a medium bowl, beat with a fork to blend. Add the mushrooms, tossing to coat with dressing.

Savory Butternut Squash Soup

Savory Butternut Squash Soup

INGREDIENTS

- 3 lbs. butternut or other winter squash
- 2 large unpeeled onions
- 1 garlic bulb
- 1/4 cup olive oil
- 2 tablespoons minced fresh thyme
- 3 cups chicken broth
- 3/4 cup coconut milk
- 3 tablespoons minced fresh parsley
- 1/2 teaspoon sea salt
- 1/2 teaspoon pepper
- Fresh thyme sprigs

STEPS

Cut squash into halves and scrape out seeds. Place cut side up in a large baking pan. Cut off tops of onion and garlic bulbs. Place cut side up in same baking pan. Brush with oil, and sprinkle with thyme. Cover tightly with foil and bake at 350 degrees for 1 1/2 to 2 hours or until vegetables are very tender. Uncover and let stand until lukewarm.

Peel squash and onions; squeeze soft garlic out of skins. Combine vegetables, broth and coconut milk. Puree in small batches in blender until smooth; transfer to a large saucepan. Add parsley, sea salt and pepper. Heat through, but do not boil. Garnish with thyme.

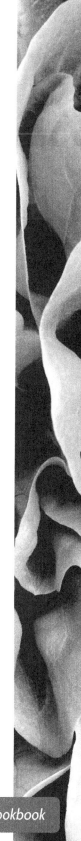

The Paleo Diet Solution Cookbook

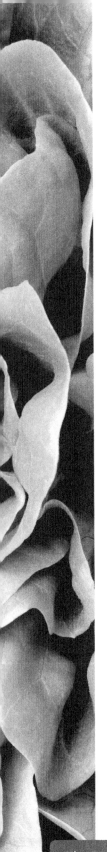

Zesty Shrimp Stuffed Avocados

INGREDIENTS

- 3 large avocados
- Juice of 1 lemon
- 1 pound cooked shelled shrimp (reserve 6 whole shrimp), coarsely chopped
- 1 hot chili pepper, peeled if fresh, seeded, washed and chopped fine
- 1 hard-cooked egg, chopped
- 2 dozen pitted black olives, sliced
- 1/3 to 1/2 cup Paleo Mayo (see next recipe)
- Ground pepper
- 3 tablespoons minced fresh cilantro

STEPS

Cut avocados in half lengthwise, pit and scoop out the flesh. Put the flesh into a bowl, then sprinkle the shells and flesh with lemon juice to prevent darkening. Mash the avocado.

Add the shrimp, hot pepper, egg and olives and mix well. Add enough mayonnaise, beginning with 1/3 cup, to bind together. Pepper to taste.

Stuff the avocado shells with this mixture. Top each with one of the reserved shrimp and sprinkle with cilantro. 6 servings.

Paleo Mayo

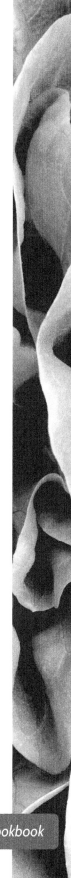

INGREDIENTS

- 1 whole egg
- 1/2 teaspoon dry mustard
- 1 cup extra virgin olive oil
- 2 tablespoons fresh lemon juice
- 1 tablespoon boiling water

STEPS

Place the egg, mustard and 1/4 cup of the oil in a blender. Turn on the motor and add the remaining 3/4 cup oil in a slow, thin stream. Add the lemon juice and water. Refrigerate.

Makes 1 1/2 cups

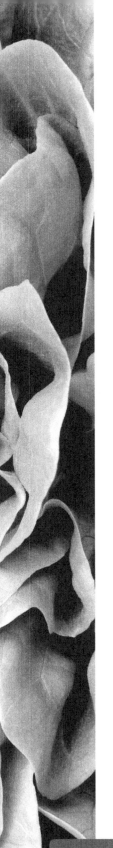

Shrimp and Shroom Antipasto

INGREDIENTS

- 1 celery rib, halved
- 1/2 small onion
- 1 sprig fresh thyme or 1 teaspoon dry
- 1/2 lemon plus 1 tablespoon fresh lemon juice
- 3 whole peppercorns, crushed
- 1/8 teaspoon hot pepper flakes
- 1/2 cup chopped tomato
- 1/8 teaspoon pepper
- 8 ounces sliced fresh mushrooms
- 12 romaine lettuce leaves
- 1 lb. medium shrimp, shelled and deveined
- 1/2 cup mayonnaise (use Paleo Mayo recipe)
- 1 tablespoon chopped fresh basil or 1/2 tsp dried

STEPS

Bring 6 cups of water to a boil with the celery, thyme, 1/2 lemon, peppercorns and hot pepper flakes. Add shrimp and cook until they just turn pink, 2-3 minutes. Drain in a colander and discard lemon. Allow to cool.

In a small bowl, combine mayo, tomato, basil, pepper and 1 tablespoon lemon juice. Beat with a fork to blend. Add mushrooms and shrimp and toss to coat. Pile salad onto lettuce leaves.

Paleo Mock Shrimp Fried Rice

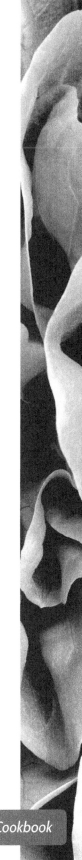

INGREDIENTS

- 1 head cauliflower
- 1 yellow onion quartered and sliced
- 1 lb. shrimp shelled and deveined and cooked
- 2 cloves garlic, minced
- 2 eggs
- 2 tablespoons safflower oil
- Salt and pepper to taste

STEPS

Chop cauliflower in food processor to a rice/couscous-like consistency. Set aside.

Sauté chopped onion and garlic in oil. Add cauliflower to skillet. Cook on high heat in order to brown "rice." Add shrimp to skillet and heat for a minute or two. Beat eggs and season with salt and pepper. Drizzle eggs into skillet and cook, stirring constantly until eggs are set.

PALEO-STYLE TUNA SALAD

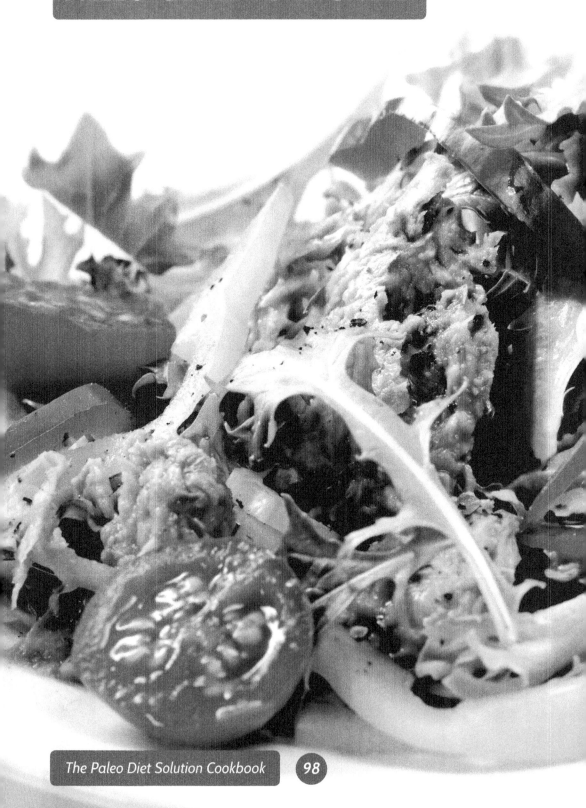

Paleo-Style Tuna Salad

INGREDIENTS

- 1 medium onion, chopped
- 2 stalks celery, chopped
- 2 tablespoons minced fresh parsley
- 1 tablespoon lemon juice
- Salt and pepper
- 2 cans albacore tuna
- 1/3 cup red pepper, chopped
- 1/3 to 1/2 cup Paleo Mayo

STEPS

Drain the tuna and mix all of the ingredients together.

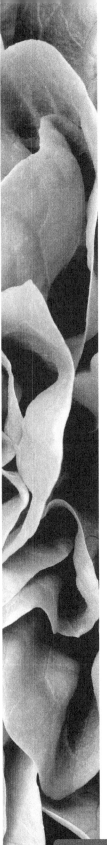

Roast Beef Salad

INGREDIENTS

- *1 celery stalk, chopped*
- *3 oz. roast beef, home cooked and shredded*
- *1 teaspoon olive oil*
- *2 teaspoons balsamic vinegar*
- *2 tablespoons Dijon mustard or Paleo Mayonnaise*
- *Romaine lettuce leaves*

STEPS

Mix the first five ingredients together and spread on lettuce leaves and roll up.

Easy Egg Drop Soup

INGREDIENTS

- 1 medium onion, diced
- 2 stalks of celery, sliced thin
- 1 tablespoon sesame oil
- 8 cups of chicken broth
- 1 teaspoon fresh ginger, grated
- 1 tablespoon wheat-free tamari sauce
- 3 tablespoons arrowroot powder
- 3 tablespoons water
- 6 eggs

STEPS

Sauté onions and celery in sesame oil over low heat until they turn soft. Stir in broth.

Add ginger and tamari sauce. Bring to a boil.

Mix arrowroot powder with water until smooth. Pour into soup and cook until thickened.

Whisk eggs and add to soup in a thin stream, stirring slowly.

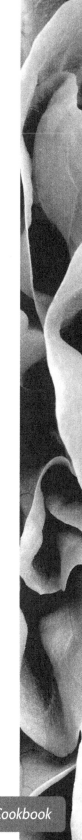

Tuscan Chicken Breasts

Tuscan Chicken Breasts

INGREDIENTS

- 4 boneless, skinless chicken breasts
- 4 tablespoons extra virgin olive oil
- Juice of 1 lemon
- 1/2 teaspoon sea salt
- 1/2 teaspoon freshly ground pepper
- 6 cloves garlic, chopped
- 1 large onion, chopped
- 1 (28-oz) can plum tomatoes, drained and chopped
- 1/2 cup pitted black olives, sliced
- 3 tablespoons fresh parsley, chopped fine (divided)
- 2 teaspoons fresh thyme, minced
- 1 teaspoon dried rosemary

STEPS

Marinate chicken in 2 tablespoons olive oil, lemon juice, sea salt and freshly ground black pepper for 30 to 60 minutes, turning often.

Preheat oven to 375 degrees.

In a large skillet, sauté garlic and onions in 2 tablespoons olive oil.

Add tomatoes and olives and sauté for 15 minutes, uncovered, stirring often.

Add 1 tablespoon parsley, rosemary and thyme, stirring to combine.

Place chicken breasts in ovenproof baking dish. Cover with sautéed mixture and sprinkle with remaining parsley.

Cover and bake for 35 to 40 minutes.

PERSONAL PALEO PIZZAS

Personal Paleo Pizzas

INGREDIENTS

- 1 cup almond flour
- 3 tablespoons almond butter
- 2 eggs, beaten
- 1/2 teaspoon sea salt
- 4 teaspoons olive oil, divided
- 1/2 cup marinara sauce
- 1/2 cup red onion, diced
- 1/2 cup fresh mushrooms, sliced
- 1 large Italian sausage, cut into 1/2-inch slices
- 2 cloves garlic, minced
- 1 red pepper, diced
- 1/2 teaspoon dried oregano
- 1/2 teaspoon fennel seed
- 1/2 teaspoon dried basil
- 1/2 cup sliced black olives

STEPS

Preheat the oven to 350 degrees.

Mix almond flour, almond butter, eggs and sea salt in a small bowl.

Grease a baking sheet with 2 teaspoons olive oil, then spread the almond mixture over it, 1/4 inch thick. Bake for 10 minutes.

Sauté the remaining olive oil, onions, mushrooms and sliced sausage in a large skillet over medium-high heat until the sausage is browned and the onions are slightly translucent. Add red pepper and garlic to skillet and cook for 1 minute, stirring constantly.

Remove the crust from the oven and cover with marinara sauce. Add the sausage and sautéed vegetables. Sprinkle with oregano, basil and fennel seed then bake for 20-30 minutes.

Remove from oven when fully cooked and top with sliced olives.

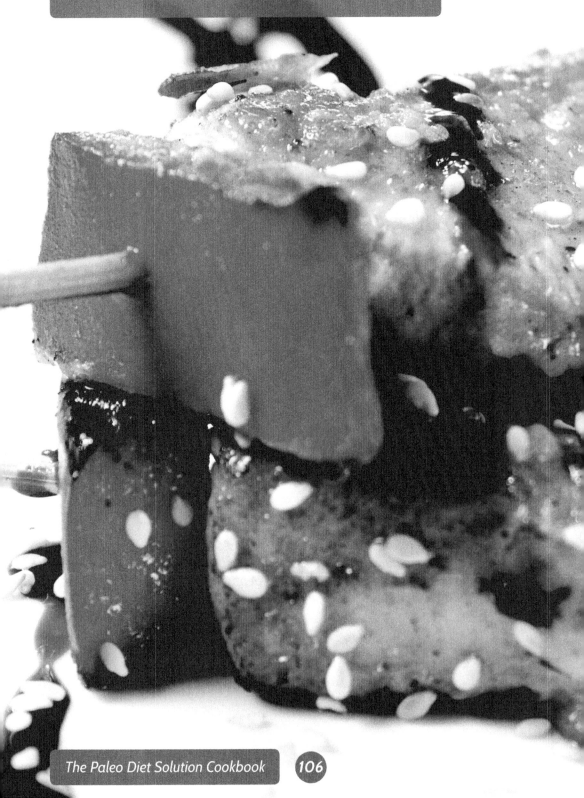

SESAME CHICKEN SKEWERS

Sesame Chicken Skewers

INGREDIENTS

Paste:
- 1/4 cup shallots
- 4 garlic cloves
- 1/4 cup fresh ginger, sliced
- 1 Serrano chili pepper, seeds removed
- 1/3 cup extra virgin olive oil

Chicken:
- 12 boneless, skinless chicken thighs cut into strips
- 1/2 teaspoon sea salt
- 1/4 teaspoon cayenne pepper

Sesame Sauce:
- 1 1/4 cups coconut milk
- 1/2 cup sesame butter
- 2 tablespoons lime juice
- 1 tablespoon fish sauce
- 1/4 teaspoon fresh ground black pepper

STEPS

In blender, puree the ginger, shallots, garlic and chili pepper. Add oil in a slow stream to make the paste. Put half the paste into a saucepan.

Put the chicken strips into a Ziploc bag with the other half of the paste and the salt and pepper. Seal the bag, pushing out the air, and massage the paste to coat all the chicken. Marinate for one hour in refrigerator.

Heat the paste in saucepan to medium-high for 3 minutes, stirring often.

Add the sauce ingredients and whisk until smooth,

Cook on low for three to four minutes until creamy.

Thread the chicken on skewers and broil for five to seven minutes, turning once. Serve with warm sauce.

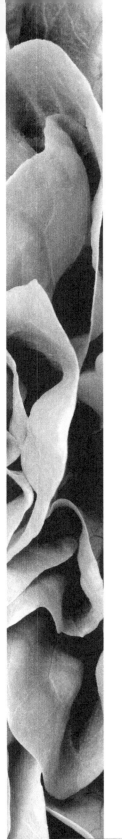

Herbed Turkey Burgers

INGREDIENTS
- 1 lb. ground turkey
- 1 cup parsley, chopped
- 1/2 cup diced onions
- 2 cloves garlic, minced
- 1 teaspoon sea salt
- 1/2 teaspoon freshly ground black pepper

STEPS
Preheat broiler.

Combine all ingredients in a bowl and mix lightly.

Divide into 4 portions and shape into patties.

Broil until cooked to desired temperature.

Paleo Hamburger or Deli Rolls

INGREDIENTS

- 4 eggs
- 4 tablespoons coconut flour
- 4 tablespoons almond flour
- 4 tablespoons coconut oil (melted)
- 1 teaspoon baking powder

STEPS

Preheat oven to 350 degrees.

In a large bowl, mix coconut flour, almond flour, baking powder and sea salt.

In a separate bowl, whisk eggs and coconut oil.

Pour egg mixture into flour mixture and combine completely.

Line a baking sheet with parchment paper, and grease the paper lightly with coconut oil.

Pour the batter onto the oiled parchment paper to make eight (3-inch diameter) pools.

Bake for 10 minutes.

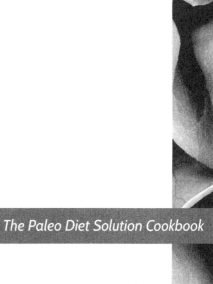

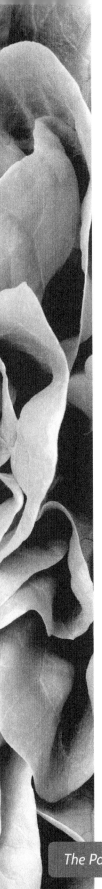

Nacho Salad

INGREDIENTS

- 1 lb. lean ground beef
- 2 tablespoons chili powder
- 1 clove garlic, minced
- 1 teaspoon cumin
- 1/2 teaspoon dried oregano
- 1/2 tsp sea salt
- 1 tablespoon olive oil
- 1 onion, diced
- 1 medium tomato, diced
- 3 romaine hearts, sliced
- 1 can black olives, sliced
- 1 avocado, cubed
- 1/4 cup minced fresh cilantro
- 1 small jar of salsa

STEPS

Brown the beef in olive oil in large skillet. Add garlic, cumin, oregano, salt and onion. Cook for three minutes on medium heat. In serving bowl toss romaine, tomato and avocado.

Add ground beef, sprinkle with olives and cilantro and serve with salsa.

Portobello Club Sandwiches

INGREDIENTS

- 4 large Portobello mushrooms
- 1/4 cup almond butter
- 1 tomato, sliced
- 1/4 cup lettuce
- 1/2 avocado sliced
- 2 slices red onion
- 1/4 lb. sliced turkey
- Cajun seasoning

STEPS

Preheat oven to 375 degrees. Remove stems from mushrooms and scrape off gills with a spoon.

Brush with almond butter and sprinkle on Cajun seasoning. Bake for 15 minutes. Place two mushroom caps on each serving plate and layer on the lettuce, tomato, turkey, red onion and avocado to make open-faced sandwiches.

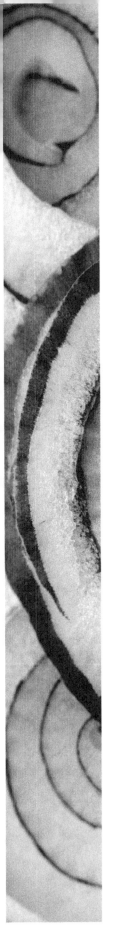

SECTION THREE

Dinner Recipes

Spicy Thai-Style Shrimp Soup

Jamaican Pepper Pot

Roasted Lebanese Chicken

Chicken Ratatouille

Citrus Marinated Flank Steak

Garlic Roasted Chicken

Sweet and Saucy Chicken Thighs

Roast Loin of Venison

Savory Roasted Rabbit

Chuck Steak Italiano

Island Style Beef Curry

Lamb with Spinach and Sweet Peppers

Caveman's Oven Fried Fish

Fast and Dill-icious Baked Salmon

Quick and Easy Shrimp Curry

Spicy Thai-Style Shrimp Soup

INGREDIENTS

- 1 tablespoon olive oil
- Shells from shrimp (see below)
- 8 cups chicken stock
- 3 stalks lemongrass, cut into 1-inch lengths
- 4 kaffir lime leaves
- 1 teaspoon lime zest
- 2 green Serrano chilies, slivered
- 2 pounds fresh shrimp, shelled (reserve shells for broth)
- 1 cup coconut milk
- 1/2 teaspoon salt
- 1 lime, juiced
- 1 red Serrano chili, slivered
- 2 tablespoons fresh cilantro, chopped
- 1 tablespoon fresh basil, chiffonade
- 3 green onions, 1/2-inch slices

STEPS

Heat the oil in a saucepan and fry the shells until they turn pink. Add the chicken stock, lemongrass, lime leaves, lime zest and green chilies. Bring to a boil, cover, reduce heat and simmer for 15 minutes.

Strain the broth through a sieve, return the liquid to a saucepan and bring to a boil.

Add the shrimp and cook them for 2-3 minutes. Reduce heat to simmer and add the coconut milk, salt and lime juice. Stir and immediately remove from heat to prevent overcooking.

Pour the soup in a serving bowl and sprinkle with red chilies, cilantro, basil and green onions.

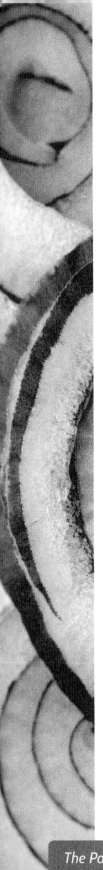

Jamaican Pepper Pot

INGREDIENTS

- 1 1/2 pounds beef round, cut into 2-inch cubes
- 3/4 pound pig's tail
- About 4 quarts water
- 1/2 pound dasheen, 1/4-inch diced
- 2 1/2 pounds fresh spinach, finely chopped
- 1 1/2 pounds kale, finely chopped
- 12 fresh okra pods, cut into small rings
- 1 hard-boiled egg, chopped
- 1 whole green Scotch bonnet pepper
- 1 large onion, chopped
- 2 garlic cloves, crushed and minced
- 3 scallions
- 4 thyme sprigs
- 1 cup coconut milk
- Salt and pepper to taste

STEPS

Put the stew meat and the pig's tail into a large soup pot and cover them with water. Bring the mixture to a boil. Boil until the meat is nearly completely cooked, then add the dasheen.

Put the spinach, kale and okra into a saucepan with a little water. Cover the pan, and cook the greens, over medium heat, for about 8 minutes.

Put the greens into a blender in batches with some broth from the meat and add the puree to the pot. Add the egg and the Scotch bonnet pepper, onion, garlic, scallions and thyme. Simmer the soup until it thickens, then add the coconut milk. Simmer the soup for 5 minutes more. Season it with salt and pepper, and serve. Serves 10.

Roasted Lebanese Chicken

INGREDIENTS

- 3/4 cup lemon juice
- 6 cloves garlic, minced
- 2 tablespoons fresh thyme, minced
- 1 tablespoon paprika
- 2 teaspoons ground cumin
- 1 teaspoon cayenne pepper
- 2 chickens split lengthwise, backbones removed and discarded
- 1 lemon, sliced
- 1/2 cup minced parsley

STEPS

Mix lemon juice, garlic, thyme, paprika, cumin and cayenne in small bowl. Place chicken in 13"x9" glass baking dish. Pour marinade over chicken and turn chicken to coat. Cover and refrigerate at least 6 hours or overnight, turning occasionally.

Preheat oven to 425 degrees. Transfer chicken and marinade to large roasting pan.

Season chicken with salt and pepper. Bake until chicken is golden brown and cooked through, basting occasionally with pan juices, about 50 min. Garnish with lemon slices and parsley.

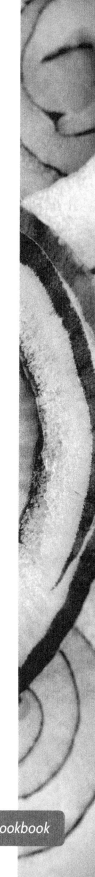

CHICKEN RATATOUILLE

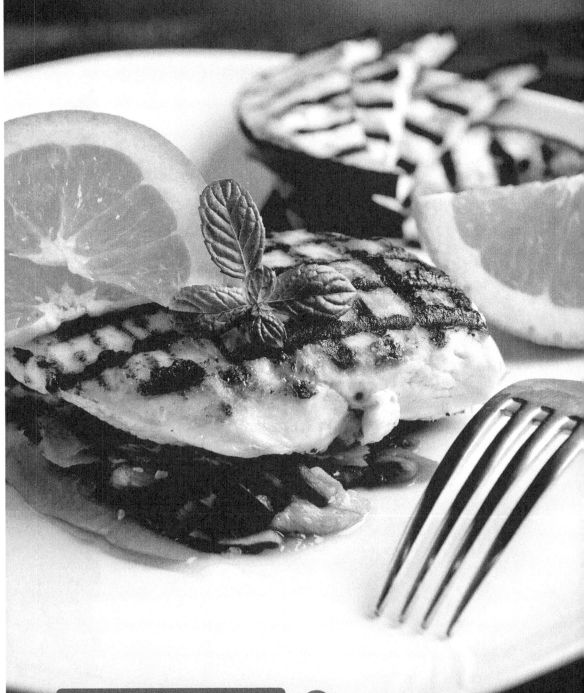

Chicken Ratatouille

INGREDIENTS

- 2 medium zucchini, cut into 2-inch pieces
- 1 red bell pepper, cut into 1-inch strips
- 1 yellow bell pepper, cut into 1-inch strips
- 1 red onion, peeled, cut into 1/4-inch slices
- 2 medium tomatoes, halved crosswise
- 4 Portobello mushroom caps, sliced thick
- 2 tablespoons olive oil
- 4 boneless skinless chicken breasts
- 1/3 cup thinly sliced fresh basil
- 1 tablespoon balsamic vinegar

STEPS

Prepare barbecue or preheat oven to 400 degrees. Place veggies in a large bowl and drizzle oil over and sprinkle generously with salt and pepper; toss to coat. Grill vegetables until tender and slightly charred. (Or oven roast until tender, about 20 minutes.) Transfer to cutting board.

Place chicken breasts in same large bowl. Turn to coat with any remaining oil in bowl. Sprinkle chicken with salt and pepper. Grill chicken, covered, until cooked through, about 6 minutes per side. Let stand 5 minutes.

Meanwhile, coarsely chop vegetables and transfer to another large bowl. Add basil and vinegar and toss to coat. Season with salt and pepper. Slice chicken crosswise into 1/2-inch-thick slices; serve with ratatouille.

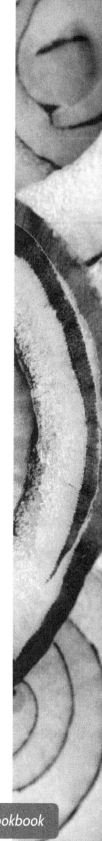

CITRUS MARINATED FLANK STEAK

Citrus Marinated Flank Steak

INGREDIENTS

- 1 (2lb.) Flank Steak
- 1 orange, juiced
- 3 limes, juiced
- 4 cloves of garlic, peeled and crushed
- 1 tablespoon brown mustard
- 1 tablespoon raspberry vinegar
- Green onion, sliced (for garnish)

STEPS

Combine orange and lime juice in a small bowl. Whisk in garlic, mustard and vinegar.

Place flank steak in a 1-gallon Ziploc bag, add marinade, and place in a refrigerator for 30 minutes to an hour.

Preheat broiler.

Broil flank steak for 6-7 minutes per side, turning once.

Slice diagonally with the grain and garnish with green onion.

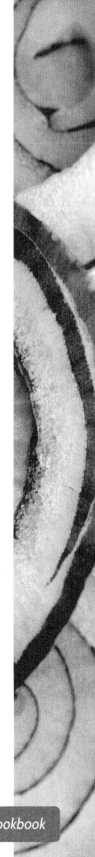

GARLIC ROASTED CHICKEN

Garlic Roasted Chicken

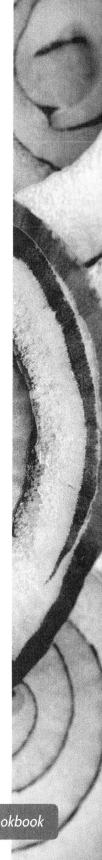

INGREDIENTS

- 1 (4-5 lb.) chicken
- 1 tablespoon ground sage
- 8 cloves garlic, peeled and sliced in half
- 1 tablespoon extra virgin olive oil
- Salt and pepper

STEPS

Preheat oven to 375 degrees. Wash chicken inside and out, pat dry with paper towels.

In a small bowl, mix together sage, oil, salt and pepper. Rub this mixture under the skin of the breast and on the skin all over the chicken. Insert half the garlic slices under the skin of the breast, drum and thigh. Put the remaining garlic slices inside the chicken. Place chicken, breast-side down, on lightly greased pan.

Roast for 30 minutes, then turn chicken breast-side up and continue roasting until internal temperature reaches 180 degrees on a meat thermometer.

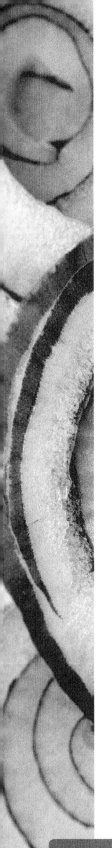

Sweet and Saucy Chicken Thighs

INGREDIENTS

- 4 tablespoons olive oil
- 1 onion, chopped
- 1/4 cup finely chopped celery
- 3 garlic cloves, minced
- 2 Granny Smith apples, cored and chopped
- 1/4 cup raisins
- 1/4 cup fresh parsley, chopped
- 1 egg, beaten
- 8 large chicken thighs
- 1 teaspoon dried tarragon

STEPS

Sauté onion, celery and garlic in 2 tablespoons oil until tender. Remove from heat and add apple, raisins, parsley and egg; mix well.

Preheat oven to 350 degrees.

Stuff apple mixture between the skin and meat. Arrange chicken pieces in a foil-lined baking dish. In a small bowl, combine the remaining olive oil with tarragon. Brush over chicken thighs.

Bake, uncovered, basting every 15 minutes, for 1 hour, until chicken is tender.

Roast Loin of Venison

INGREDIENTS

- 4 pounds boneless loin of venison, at room temperature
- 2 tablespoons extra virgin olive oil
- 1 teaspoon freshly ground pepper
- 1/2 teaspoon finely chopped juniper berries
- 1 teaspoon sea salt

STEPS

Preheat the oven to 400 degrees. Rub the venison with the olive oil, salt, pepper and juniper.

Set the loin on a rack in a roasting pan and roast, basting frequently with the pan juices, until medium-rare, about 30 minutes. It should register 130 degrees on a meat thermometer.

Cover the venison loosely with foil and set aside for 10 to 15 minutes before carving. Slice the venison thinly.

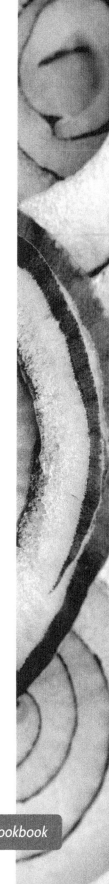

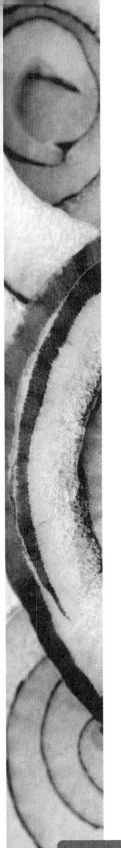

Savory Roasted Rabbit

INGREDIENTS

- 2 tablespoons olive oil
- 1 rabbit (about 2 1/2 lb.), cut into pieces
- Salt & pepper to taste
- 1 onion sliced
- 3 cloves garlic; minced
- 3/4 cup chicken stock
- 1 teaspoon dried rosemary
- 2 tablespoons dried parsley
- 1 bay leaf

STEPS

Preheat the oven to 350 degrees.

Brown the rabbit pieces in a skillet in batches in oil for about 5 to 7 minutes per side, sprinkling with salt and pepper. Place the browned rabbit into a shallow baking pan.

Add the onion to the skillet and cook over low heat to soften. Add the garlic and cook 2 minutes more, stirring. Add broth and bay leaf and bring to a boil, deglazing the skillet. Reduce the heat; add the rosemary and parsley. Cook sauce for 2 minutes longer.

Pour the sauce over the rabbit and bake for 45 minutes. To serve, place rabbit pieces on a serving platter and pour all remaining pan juices over top.

Chuck Steak Italiano

INGREDIENTS

- 1 beef chuck steak, cut 1 inch thick, 1 1/2 to 2 pounds
- 1 onion, sliced
- 1 (14-oz) can Italian plum tomatoes, drained and chopped
- 1 teaspoon dried oregano
- 1 teaspoon dried rosemary
- 4 garlic cloves, chopped
- 1 teaspoon red pepper flakes
- 2 tablespoons olive oil

STEPS

Preheat oven to 350 degrees. Place steak in a 9"x13" glass baking dish. In a bowl, combine all other ingredients.

Spread over top of steak. Bake steak uncovered 45 minutes to 1 hour, or until tender.

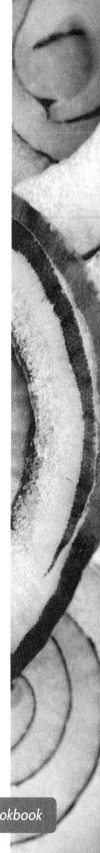

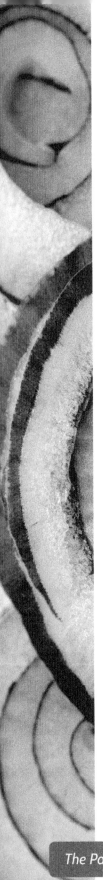

Island Style Beef Curry

INGREDIENTS

Spice Paste:
- 4 to 8 large dried New Mexico chilies
- 4 lemongrass stalks
- 1/2 cup onions, chopped
- 6 cloves garlic, peeled
- 2 teaspoons coriander
- 2 teaspoons cumin
- 1 tablespoon fresh ginger, grated
- 3 tablespoons fish sauce
- 1 teaspoon turmeric
- 1 teaspoon black pepper
- 1/2 cup water

Stew:
- 3 lb. boneless chuck, trimmed and cut into 1 1/2-inch cubes
- 1 (13.5-oz) can unsweetened coconut milk
- Zest from 1 lime
- 2 whole star anise
- 1 cinnamon stick
- 1 bay leaf
- 1 tablespoon tamarind paste

STEPS

Cover the chilies with very hot water and soak until soft, about 45 minutes. Drain, stem, seed and chop chilies. Cut off the bottom 4 inches from the lemongrass stalks. Chop and transfer to food processor. Add onions, garlic, coriander, cumin, ginger, black pepper and turmeric and process until finely ground.

Add 1/2 cup water, chilies and fish sauce. Process to paste.

Mix beef and spice paste in slow cooker. Stir in coconut milk, lime zest, star anise, cinnamon, bay leaf and tamarind. Press meat down completely to submerge. Cook stew on low heat until meat is very tender, 4 1/2-5 hours. Spoon excess from surface of stew before serving. Remove bay leaf, star anise and cinnamon stick.

Lamb With Spinach and Sweet Peppers

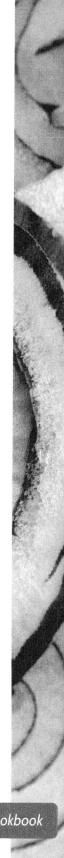

INGREDIENTS

- 3 lb. boneless leg of lamb, cut into 1 1/2-inch pieces
- 1/2 tsp pepper
- 3 Tbsp olive oil
- 4 garlic cloves, chopped
- 2 cups hot water
- 3 Tbsp chopped fresh parsley
- 2 large red bell peppers, cut into 1 1/2- to 2-inch pieces
- 1 bag prewashed fresh spinach
- 1 lemon sliced

STEPS

Season lamb with 1/4 tsp pepper. In a large frying pan heat oil over high heat.

Add lamb and cook, turning frequently, 3-5 minutes, or until browned on all sides.

Add garlic, water and remaining 1/4 tsp pepper. Bring to a boil, reduce heat to medium and cook partially covered 30 minutes. Uncover and cook 10 minutes longer, or until lamb is fork tender.

Add parsley and red peppers to pan. Cook 10 minutes, or until peppers are just tender. Steam spinach while meat is cooking and serve meat on a bed of spinach garnished with lemon slices.

Caveman's Oven Fried Fish

Caveman's Oven Fried Fish

INGREDIENTS

- *2 flounder filets, defrosted*
- *1 egg*
- *1 tablespoon water*
- *1/3 to 1/2 cup nut flour*
- *1 teaspoon paprika*
- *Fresh ground black pepper to taste*

STEPS

Whisk egg and water in shallow bowl. On a plate, mix nut flour, paprika and pepper.

Dip filets in egg and then roll in nut flour. Let fish stand on waxed paper while oven heats to 375 degrees. Lightly oil a baking dish with olive oil and bake for 12 minutes or until fish flakes and meat is opaque.

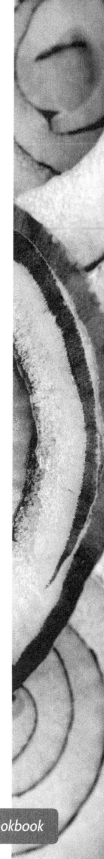

FAST AND DILL-ICIOUS BAKED SALMON

Fast and Dill-icious Baked Salmon

INGREDIENTS

- 4 (6 oz.) salmon fillets
- 1/2 teaspoon salt
- 1/4 teaspoon pepper
- 2 tablespoons chopped fresh dill
- 4 lemon slices
- 3 chopped shallots
- 1 chopped garlic clove
- 2 tablespoons olive oil
- 2 bags prewashed spinach
- 1 cup lightly packed basil
- 1/4 cup broth or stock

STEPS

Preheat oven to 350 degrees.

Season both sides of filets with salt, pepper and dill. Place salmon fillets on baking pan.

Place a lemon slice on each filet. Bake at 350 degrees for 15 minutes.

Sauté shallots and chopped garlic clove in olive oil until translucent, add spinach, basil and stock. Cover and steam until greens are wilted. Serve salmon on a bed of spinach.

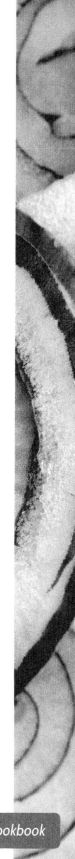

The Paleo Diet Solution Cookbook

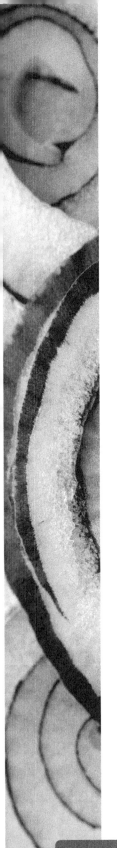

Quick and Easy Shrimp Curry

INGREDIENTS

- 2 tablespoons extra virgin olive oil
- 1 red onion, sliced thin and quartered
- 1 (8 oz.) can tomato sauce
- 2 teaspoons grated fresh ginger
- 4 cloves garlic, minced
- 1 teaspoon cumin
- 1 teaspoon coriander
- 1/2 teaspoon turmeric
- 1/2 teaspoon freshly ground black pepper
- 10 oz. frozen shelled shrimp, defrosted
- 1/4 cup fresh cilantro, chopped
- 1 tablespoon lime juice

STEPS

Heat oil and sauté onion at low temperature until golden. Add tomato sauce, ginger, garlic and spices. Bring to simmer. Add a little water if too thick. Add shrimp to sauce. Simmer 3 minutes or until shrimp is cooked through. Add a little lime juice just before serving and sprinkle with cilantro.

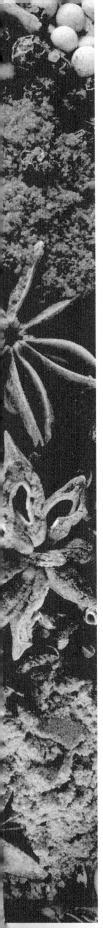

Dessert Recipes

Paleo-Friendly Coconut Custard

INGREDIENTS

- 1 (14-oz) can coconut milk
- 1/4 cup honey
- 1/2 teaspoon nutmeg
- 1/2 teaspoon cinnamon
- 2 eggs

STEPS

Preheat oven to 325 degrees.

Whisk eggs until light then add the rest of the ingredients. Pour into custard cups and place cups in large baking dish. Fill with a water bath halfway to the top of the custard cups.

Bake for 30 minutes or until a knife inserted in the center of the custard comes out clean.

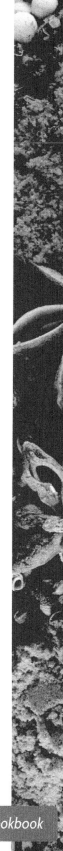

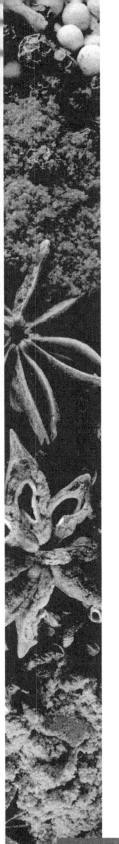

Citrus Roasted Bananas

INGREDIENTS

- 4 bananas peeled
- 1 teaspoon grated orange rind
- 2 tablespoons pure maple syrup
- 1 tablespoon lemon juice
- 1/8 teaspoon salt
- 1 teaspoon cinnamon
- 1/2 teaspoon mace
- 1 tablespoon melted coconut oil

STEPS

Cut each banana in half lengthwise. Arrange banana slices in a baking dish.

Mix syrup, juice and oil together and drizzle evenly over bananas. Mix salt, cinnamon and mace together and sprinkle over bananas evenly. Bake at 350 degrees for 30 minutes. Sprinkle with orange rind before serving.

Pumpkin Custard

INGREDIENTS

- 1/2 cup honey
- 1/2 teaspoon salt
- 1 teaspoon cinnamon
- 1 teaspoon ginger
- 1/4 teaspoon ground cloves
- 1/2 teaspoon allspice
- 2 eggs
- 1 (15-oz.) can pumpkin
- 1 1/2 cups coconut milk

STEPS

Preheat oven to 375 degrees.

In a large bowl, whisk eggs until light. Add everything but the pumpkin and mix well.

Add half the pumpkin and mix until smooth, then add the rest. Bake in a soufflé pan for 35 to 45 minutes or until a knife inserted in the center comes out clean.

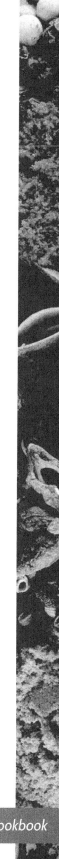

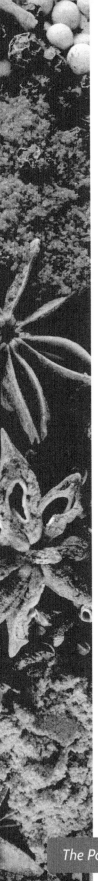

Autumn Harvest Compote

INGREDIENTS

- 2 cups fresh squeezed orange juice
- 1 cup pineapple juice
- 1 teaspoon cinnamon
- 1 teaspoon ginger
- 1/2 teaspoon ground cloves
- 1/2 cup dried cranberries
- 1 cup raisins
- 1 cup prunes
- 1 cup figs
- 2 cups dried apricots
- 1/2 cup slivered almonds

STEPS

Heat juices and spices slowly until almost boiling. Add all the fruits and simmer for about 10 minutes. Serve warm sprinkled with almonds.

Italian Chestnut Cake

INGREDIENTS

* 10 1/2 oz. chestnut flour
* 1/4 cup raw honey
* 2 tablespoons dried cherries, chopped
* 3 sprigs fresh rosemary
* 1/2 teaspoon sea salt
* 1 teaspoon nutmeg
* Tepid water
* 3 tablespoons extra virgin olive oil

STEPS

Preheat oven to 375 degrees and grease a 12" cake pan.

Sift flour, salt and nutmeg into a bowl and begin to whisk in warm water until the batter is thick and smooth. Add the cherries and oil and mix well. Pour into pan and lay rosemary across top. Bake for 30 to 40 minutes, checking in the last 10 minutes to make sure it does not get too dark or too dry.

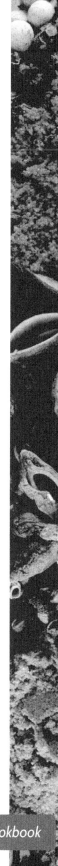

Macaroons

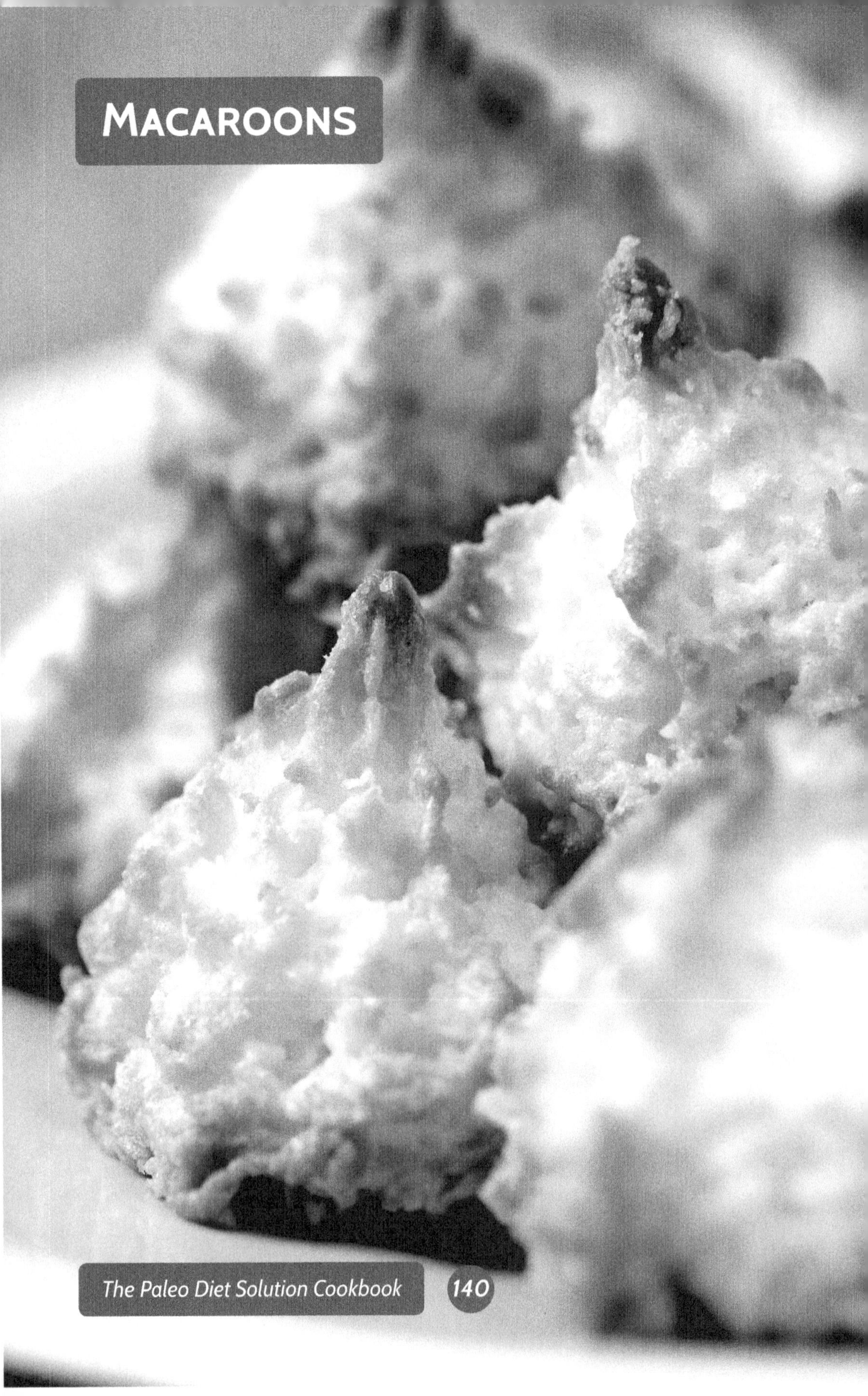

Macaroons

INGREDIENTS

- 2 2/3 cups unsweetened shredded coconut
- 1 cup sliced raw almonds
- 1/4 teaspoon salt
- 1/4 cup honey
- 5 egg whites

STEPS

Preheat oven to 325 degrees. Grease two large cookie sheets.

Measure coconut, almonds and honey and salt into bowl and mix completely. Stir in egg whites and blend well. Drop by tablespoonful 2 inches apart. Bake 20 to 25 minutes until lightly browned.

Cool on wire racks and store in tightly covered container. Makes about 2 dozen.

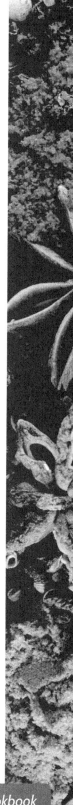

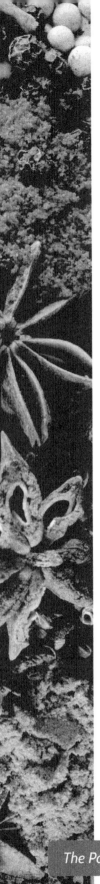

Carrot Cake

INGREDIENTS

- 6 eggs, separated
- 1/2 cup pure maple syrup
- 1 1/2 cups carrots, cooked and pureed
- 1 tablespoon grated orange rind
- 1 tablespoon frozen, concentrated orange juice
- 3 cups almond flour
- 1/2 teaspoon salt
- 1 teaspoon nutmeg

STEPS

Preheat oven to 325 degrees and grease a 9" springform pan.

Beat egg yolks and honey until light. Stir in carrots, orange zest, juice, flour and seasonings. Beat the egg whites until stiff and fold in gently.

Bake 45 to 50 minutes or until a toothpick inserted into the center comes out clean. Let cool for 20 minutes before removing from pan.

Pastry

INGREDIENTS

- 2 1/2 cups almond flour
- 2/3 cup shortening
- 1/2 teaspoon salt
- 1/3 cup ice cold water

STEPS

Preheat oven to 450 degrees.

Combine flour and salt in a bowl and cut shortening in with a pastry blender until crumbs are the size of peas. Add water slowly until pastry holds together when pressed between your fingers, Do not add more water than necessary. Roll dough into a ball. Handling as little as possible, roll out on a floured board 1/8 inch thick and one inch larger than the diameter of your pie pan. Press gently into the pan, trim edges and prick all over with a fork. Bake 12 to 15 minutes until golden brown.

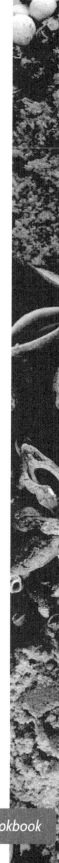

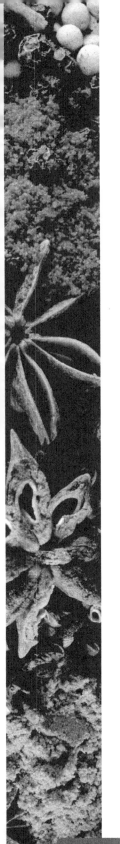

Almond Cookies

INGREDIENTS

- 2 1/2 cups honey
- 2 cups ground almonds
- 2 1/2 cups almond flour
- 1 teaspoon nutmeg
- 1 teaspoon ginger
- 1/2 teaspoon salt
- 1/2 cup dried cherries, chopped

STEPS

Preheat oven to 350 degrees. Lightly grease cookie sheets.

Sift together almond flour, nutmeg, ginger and salt. Stir in ground almonds until well mixed. Warm honey if it is thick or cold. Pour honey into a large bowl and gradually stir in flour mixture. Add cherries and mix evenly. Drop by teaspoonfuls and bake for about 10 minutes. Makes about 4 dozen cookies.

Pumpkin Pie With Hazelnut Crust

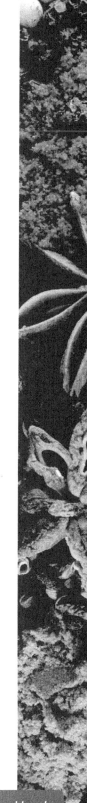

INGREDIENTS

Crust:

- *1 cup hazelnuts*
- *1 cup chestnut flour*
- *1 teaspoon pure vanilla extract*
- *1/4 cup coconut milk*
- *1/4 teaspoon salt*

Filling:

- *1 1/2 cups cooked pumpkin*
- *2/3 cup pure maple syrup*
- *1 teaspoon pure vanilla extract*
- *1 teaspoon cinnamon*
- *1 teaspoon ginger*
- *1/2 teaspoon nutmeg*
- *1 teaspoon allspice*
- *4 teaspoons arrowroot*

STEPS

Preheat oven to 350 degrees. In food processor, grind hazelnuts to a fine meal, then add the remaining ingredients and process to combine. Press the mixture into an 8" pie pan. Bake 10 to 12 minutes until light brown, being careful not to burn it.

Put all the filling ingredients into a bowl and blend with a hand mixer until smooth. Pour into the prepared pie crust and bake for 30 minutes until the filling is firm. Serve cool.

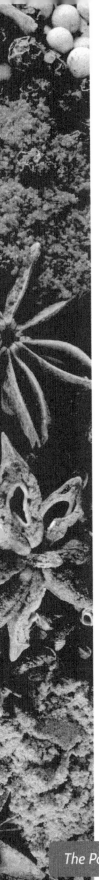

Apple Pie With Pecan-Walnut Crust

INGREDIENTS

Crust:
- *1/4 cup pecans*
- *1/4 cup walnuts*
- *4 large dates*

Filling:
- *2 Granny Smith apples peeled, cored and quartered*
- *1/2 teaspoon cinnamon*
- *1/2 teaspoon nutmeg*
- *1 teaspoon lemon juice*

STEPS

Mix crust ingredients in a food processor and press evenly into bottom and sides of pie pan.

Put all filling ingredients in food processor and chop coarsely. Spread into pie crust and serve.

Miami Ice

INGREDIENTS

- 4 large mangoes, peeled, pitted and sliced
- 1/3 cup fresh lime juice
- Zest of 1 lime
- 1 cup orange juice
- 1/4 cup honey

STEPS

In a food processor, whip all ingredients until smooth. Freeze for 2 hours until firm.

Break into chunks and beat with hand mixer and freeze again. Repeat this process twice and freeze again for at least an hour before serving.

Strawberry Sunshine Pie

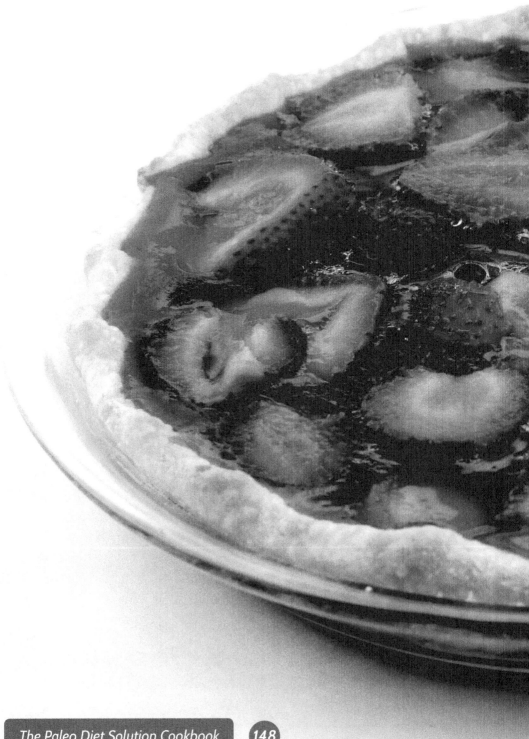

Strawberry Sunshine Pie

INGREDIENTS

- 3 pints fresh, ripe strawberries
- 5 pitted dates
- 2 bananas
- 1 1/2 tablespoons fresh lemon juice
- 1/2 teaspoon almond extract
- Prepared pie crust

STEPS

*Put 8 hulled strawberries, dates, sliced bananas, lemon juice and al-
mond extract into blender and puree. Hull and slice remaining strawberries, reserving a few choice berries for garnish. Layer the sliced berries in rounds in the prepared crust.*

*Pour puree evenly over the berries, add the garnish, cover with saran
wrap and refrigerate for at least an hour before serving.*

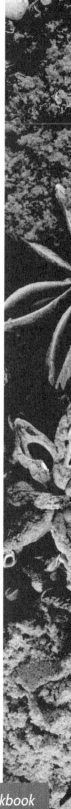

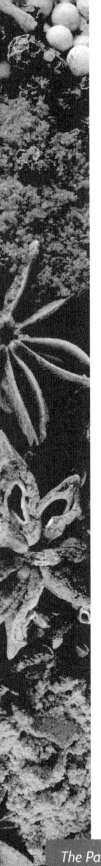

Apple Raisin Cookies

INGREDIENTS

- 2 cups almonds, soaked in water for 2 hours and peeled
- 1 cup walnuts, soaked in water for 2 hours
- 2 tart apples, grated
- 2 bananas
- 1/2 cup dates, chopped
- 1 cup raisins
- 1 teaspoon cinnamon
- 1 tablespoon sesame oil

STEPS

Process almonds, walnuts and bananas in a food processor until roughly chopped.

In bowl, mix all ingredients together well. Using a dehydrator with a Teflex sheet on the trays, form the mixture into small round cookies and place close together on the sheets. Dehydrate for about 4 hours at 105 degrees. Turn cookies over and remove the sheets from the trays. Dehydrate for another 4 hours.

Watermelon Freeze

INGREDIENTS

- 4 cups seeded and cubed watermelon
- 2 cups cubed cantaloupe
- 1 cup orange juice
- 1/4 cup mint leaves

STEPS

Puree the melons and mint in a food processor with the orange juice. Pour into small paper cups or popsicle molds. Insert sticks and freeze until firm.

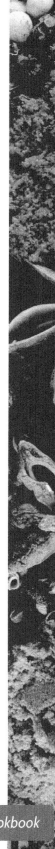

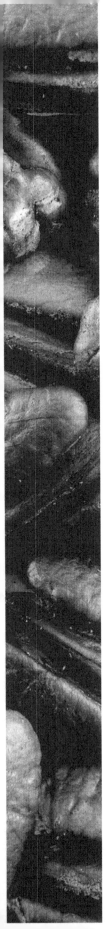

Snack Recipes

Tropical Fruit Bites

INGREDIENTS

- 1/2 cup honey
- 2 tablespoons lemon juice
- 1/2 teaspoon cinnamon
- 4 bananas
- 1 cup shredded coconut

STEPS

Whisk honey, lemon juice and cinnamon in small shallow bowl. Peel and cut bananas in 1-inch diagonal slices. Dip each piece in honey and lemon and roll in shredded coconut until coated on both sides. Chill on a nonstick baking sheet until serving time.

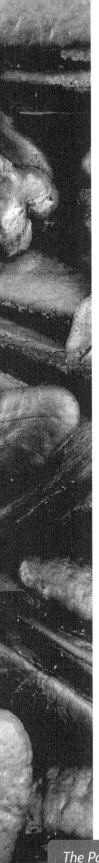

Sweet Treat Nuts

INGREDIENTS

- 2 cups fresh almonds
- 1 cup pecans
- 1 cup walnuts
- 2 egg whites
- 1 teaspoon salt
- 1/2 cup pure maple syrup
- 2 teaspoons cinnamon
- 2 teaspoons oil

STEPS

Preheat oven to 375 degrees and oil a large baking pan.

In a large bowl, mix egg, salt, syrup and cinnamon. Add nuts and toss with oil until all are coated. Spread nuts in a single layer on prepared pan and bake for 15 to 20 minutes, stirring frequently to prevent burning. Allow to cool and then store in an airtight container.

Baba Ganoush (Eggplant and Tahini)

INGREDIENTS

- 1 large eggplant
- 1/2 cup roasted red pepper, diced
- 1/4 cup fresh lemon juice
- 1/2 cup sesame butter
- 4 cloves garlic, crushed in garlic press
- 1 1/2 teaspoons of salt
- Fresh ground black pepper to taste
- 1/4 cup fresh parsley, minced
- 1 tablespoon olive oil

STEPS

Preheat oven to 450 degrees.

Cut eggplant in half but do not peel. Place face down on oiled baking sheet.

Bake for 15 minutes or until soft. Remove from oven and allow to cool.

Using oven mitts and a sharp spoon, scrape out eggplant flesh and chop fine.

Add the red pepper and mix well. In a small bowl whisk together the lemon juice, sesame butter, garlic, salt, pepper and parsley. Stir into eggplant and mix well. Serve warm with vegetable crudités.

Spicy Guacamole

Spicy Guacamole

INGREDIENTS

- 4 large ripe avocados peeled and diced
- 1 red onion, minced
- 4 garlic cloves, crushed
- 1 jalapeño pepper, seeds and pith removed, chopped fine
- 1/2 cup fresh cilantro, chopped
- 2 limes, juiced
- 1 teaspoon sea salt
- 1/2 teaspoon red pepper flakes

STEPS

Mash avocado and lime juice roughly with a fork. Add remaining ingredients and mix well. Serve immediately or place saran wrap directly on guacamole and refrigerate for a short time.

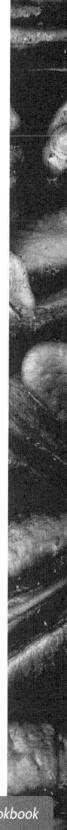

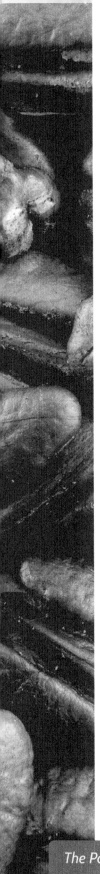

Crispy Cinnamon Apple Chips

INGREDIENTS
- 2 cups unsweetened apple cider
- 2 cinnamon sticks
- 2 Granny Smith apples

STEPS

Preheat oven to 250 degrees. In a saucepan bring cider and cinnamon to a low boil.

Core but don't peel the apples. Slice in 1/8-inch rounds.

Simmer apple slices for about 5 minutes until they become translucent.

Drain slices in a colander and pat dry. Arrange apples on cake racks without overlapping. Bake 30 to 40 minutes until apples are light brown and almost dry. Cool completely before storing in an airtight container.

Easy Mushroom Pate

INGREDIENTS

- 2 tablespoons extra virgin olive oil
- 1/3 cup onions, finely chopped
- 1/3 cup carrots, shredded
- 1/3 cup celery, finely chopped
- 2 cups fresh mushrooms, finely chopped
- 2 cloves garlic, minced
- 1 tablespoon dried parsley
- 1 teaspoon dried thyme
- Salt and pepper to taste

STEPS

In a large skillet, sauté all the ingredients, stirring frequently until any liquid has reduced, about 15 to 20 minutes. Process in a food processor until mixture is smooth and spreadable. Refrigerate until serving.

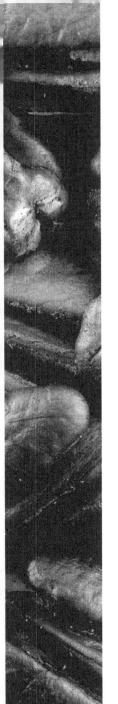

Tropi-cool Banana Treats

INGREDIENTS

- *1 banana*
- *2 tablespoons almond butter*
- *1/4 cup shredded, unsweetened coconut*

STEPS

Spread nut butter on outside of banana, roll in coconut and freeze.

Spicy Pecans

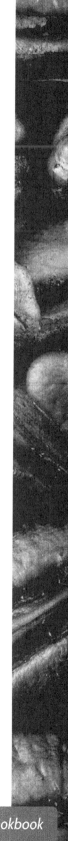

INGREDIENTS

- 4 teaspoons cinnamon
- 2 teaspoons ground ginger
- 1 teaspoon nutmeg
- 1/2 teaspoon ground cayenne
- 3 egg whites
- 1/2 cup honey
- 5 cups pecans
- Olive oil

STEPS

Preheat oven to 350 degrees.

In a large bowl, whisk egg whites until frothy. Add honey and whisk until combined. Add spices and mix in well. Add nuts to the bowl and toss until all are evenly coated. Place in one layer on oiled baking sheet and bake for 20 minutes, stirring once until golden.

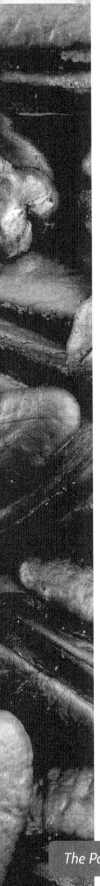

Georgia Peach Pops

INGREDIENTS

- 6 peaches, peeled and diced
- 2 bananas, sliced
- 1 can coconut milk
- 2 tablespoons fresh lemon juice
- 2 teaspoons grated fresh ginger

STEPS

Puree all ingredients in blender, in batches if necessary. Pour into popsicle molds or the smallest Dixie cups and freeze until firm.

Homemade Beef Jerky

INGREDIENTS

For each pound of meat:
- 1 teaspoon salt
- 2 teaspoons freshly ground black pepper
- 2 teaspoons chili powder
- 2 teaspoons garlic powder
- 2 teaspoons onion powder

STEPS

Mix seasonings together well in a small bowl. Rub evenly onto meat and pound in with a mallet. Cut beef into strips and lay on a rack in a roasting pan to catch drips. Set oven at 150 degrees and prop door open. Bake approximately 8 hours until the meat is dry and brittle.

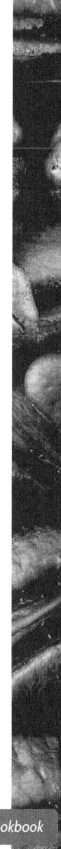

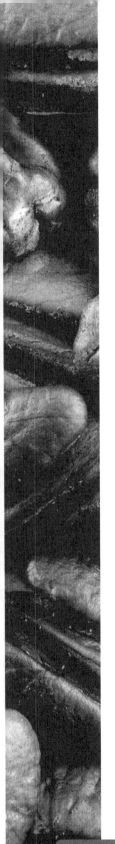

Paleo Trail Mix

INGREDIENTS

- 1 cup sunflower seeds
- 1 cup pepitas (pumpkin seeds)
- 1 cup almonds
- 1 cup Spicy Pecans (see previous recipe)
- 1 cup raisins
- 1 cup plantain chips

STEPS

Mix together in a large bowl. Measure out 1/4-cup servings and store in snack-size Ziploc bags.

Strawberry Fruit Rolls

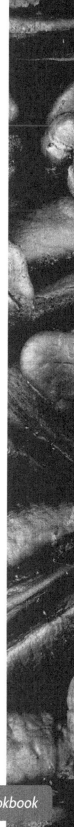

INGREDIENTS

- *4 cups fresh strawberries*
- *2 tablespoons honey*
- *1 tablespoon fresh lemon juice*

STEPS

Wash, hull and halve the strawberries and place in saucepan with honey and lemon.

Bring just to a boil, then cool and puree in blender. Pour on to nonstick cookie sheet in a 1/8-inch layer. Bake in oven and the lowest heat setting for about six hours until it becomes leathery. Cut into strips and roll up.

Store in tightly wrapped saran wrap.

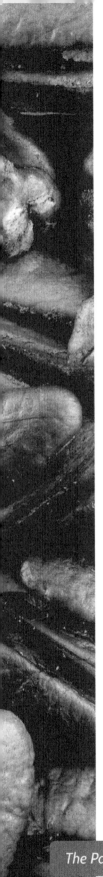

Kale Chips

INGREDIENTS

* 1 bunch kale
* 2 tablespoons olive oil
* Cajun seasoned salt

STEPS

Preheat oven to 350 degrees.

Wash kale and spin dry in salad spinner. With knife or kitchen shears cut out the thick ribs of the leaves and cut into 2-inch pieces. In large bowl, drizzle kale with olive oil and toss until evenly coated. Spread out on baking sheet and sprinkle with seasoned salt. Bake for 10 to 15 minutes until slightly crispy.

Sesame Glazed Fruit Skewers

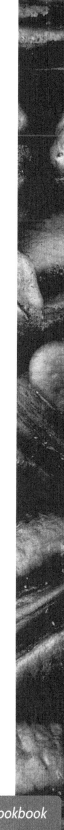

INGREDIENTS

- *1/2 cup sesame butter*
- *1/2 cup honey*
- *2 tablespoons lemon juice*
- *1 tablespoon sesame seeds*
- *2 bananas cut into 2-inch pieces*
- *2 Fuji apples, cored and cut into 2-inch wedges*
- *1 seedless orange unpeeled, cut in half rounds*
- *1/4 cup shredded coconut*
- *Bamboo skewers soaked in water*

STEPS

Preheat broiler.

In small bowl, combine sesame butter, honey, lemon juice and sesame seeds.

Thread fruits on to skewers, brush with sauce and sprinkle with coconut. Broil for two minutes on each side and serve hot.

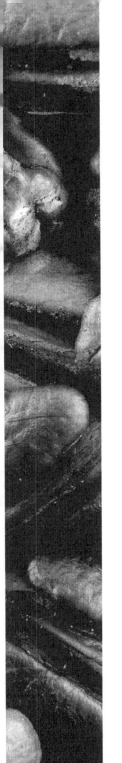

Florida Crab Dip

INGREDIENTS

- 1 cup crab claw meat, picked over to remove bits of shell
- 1/4 cup red pepper, diced fine
- 1/3 cup onion, diced fine
- 1/4 cup celery, diced fine
- 1/4 cup parsley, chopped
- 1/2 teaspoon red pepper flakes
- Dash of cayenne pepper
- 2 tablespoons fresh lemon juice
- 1/2 cup Paleo Mayo (see previous recipe)

STEPS

In a bowl, mix crab meat with lemon juice. Add all ingredients except Mayo and toss to distribute evenly. Add Mayo and stir to combine. Keep refrigerated until serving.

CPSIA information can be obtained at www.ICGtesting.com
Printed in the USA
LVOW03s1402190314

378088LV00006B/26/P

9 780615 598802